The Property of
Library Services
Hafan Derwen
Carmarthen

An Introduction to Clinical Research in Psychiatry

An Introduction to Clinical Research in Psychiatry

DAN G. BLAZER, M.D., Ph.D.
JUDITH C. HAYS, R.N., Ph.D.

New York   Oxford
OXFORD UNIVERSITY PRESS
1998

Oxford University Press

Oxford   New York
Athens   Auckland   Bangkok   Bogota
Bombay   Buenos Aires   Calcutta   Cape Town
Dar es Salaam   Delhi   Florence   Hong Kong   Istanbul
Karachi   Kuala Lumpur   Madras   Madrid
Melbourne   Mexico City   Nairobi   Paris
Singapore   Taipei   Tokyo   Toronto   Warsaw

and associated companies in
Berlin   Ibadan

Copyright © 1998 by Oxford University Press

Published by Oxford University Press, Inc.
198 Madison Avenue, New York, New York 10016

Oxford is a registered trademark of Oxford University Press

Library of Congress Cataloging-in-Publication Data
Blazer, Dan G. (Dan German), 1944–
An introduction to clinical research in psychiatry /
Dan G. Blazer, Judith C. Hays.
p.   cm.   Includes bibliographical references and index.
ISBN 0-19-510213-4
1. Psychiatry—Research—Methodology.
I. Hays, Judith C.   II. Title.
[DNLM: 1. Evaluation Studies.
2. Psychiatry.   3. Causality.
WM   20 B645 1998]
RC337.B58   1998   616.89′0072—dc21
DNLM/DC for Library of Congress   97-22573

9 8 7 6 5 4 3 2 1

Printed in the United States of America
on acid-free paper

With gratitude to our teachers,

Berton H. Kaplan, Ph.D.
and
W. Douglas Thompson, Ph.D.

PREFACE

This book is truly an introduction. For many clinicians and residents, it should provide a useful and sufficient overview of epidemiologic methods. After reading it, those who intend to do psychiatric research should naturally progress to more advanced volumes in epidemiology, biostatistics, or clinical-trial methodology. We have provided neither a systematic nor a comprehensive review of community-based epidemiologic studies, case-control studies, or clinical trials in psychiatry. Rather, we describe in simple terms the methods employed in the most common research designs, using illustrations from published studies to highlight the problems encountered by clinicians undertaking patient-oriented research in psychiatry. The types of studies reviewed are single subject design, description studies (such as case registers and population based surveys), community studies, cohort studies, and case-control studies. Clinical studies of screening and diagnostic tests and population genetic studies are considered with special attention to the analysis and interpretation of their results. The book concludes with an overview of analytic strategies used across study designs.

The book's format should enable readers to learn basic research methods with virtually no background in this area. Many residents, junior faculty, and community-based psychiatrists receive little, if any, research training. They often read journal reports of studies by skimming the abstract, introduction, and conclusions of a paper with little understanding of the methodology used to study a problem and derive conclusions from that study. This book has been written to encourage clinicians to gain direct experience of study design; it does this by using examples from the literature and supplying a problem set at the end of each chapter. The reader who follows the examples and does the problem sets should, we believe, gain an ability to evaluate journal papers.

The book's focus is on clinical research in which the patient (or subject) is the unit of analysis. The reader may therefore be surprised to find many references to community-based epidemiological studies. Our belief is that these community-based studies are not only an essential foundation for understanding clinical research but also provide excellent examples of research methods that can be applied to studies where the patient is the unit of analysis.

Though the book deals with "psychiatric research," we believe it is applicable not only to psychiatrists but also to psychologists, nurses, social workers, and other health care professionals who work in mental health centers, psychiatric hospitals, and psychiatric ambulatory care settings. The research strategies and problems we describe are common to all mental health disciplines.

This book derives in part from a course we have taught in the School of Medicine at Duke University for the past three years. We have been especially pleased with the progress medical students have made, using an interactive/problem-based approach to learning research methodology and the evaluation of research findings. The students work in small groups, complete assigned readings, and attend a series of lectures. The ideal setting for using the book may be a seminar series in research methodology for clinicians who have little or no experience with clinical research. In our own course, we have found it useful as a concluding exercise for each participant to critique an area that is somewhat controversial in clinical research by reviewing four to five studies which provide conflicting results, summarizing those studies in terms of methodological bias, and drawing conclusions about what is currently known and what studies should be initiated to clarify unknowns. Nevertheless, because all readers will not be taking courses in clinical research, we have written the book so that clinicians can easily work through it on their own.

Finally, we wish to thank Elizabeth P. Flint, Ph.D., for formatting; Jennifer Riley for typing much of the manuscript; and Jeffrey House, our editor at Oxford University Press.

Durham, North Carolina   D.G.B.
October 1997   J.C.H.

CONTENTS

III   ANALYSIS AND INTERPRETATION OF RESULTS

I

BACKGROUND

1

CAUSAL INFERENCE

OBJECTIVES

- To describe the hierarchy of evidence that supports a cause–effect relationship between a risk factor and a psychiatric disorder.
- To evaluate the specific contribution of individual studies to supporting the cause–effect relationship.
- To recognize the nature of the causal relationship—whether the risk factor is predisposing, enabling, precipitative, and/or reinforcing.
- To examine the logic of causal inference.

CASE EXAMPLE

Paykel et al. compared 185 depressed patients from both inpatient and ambulatory care settings with 185 community-based controls matched for gender, age, marital status, race/ethnicity and social class (Paykel et al., 1969). The diagnosis was based on a persistent abnormal depressed mood accompanied by other symptoms of depression such as sleep disturbance. Patients were excluded if they were also diagnosed with schizophrenia, alcoholism, or drug addiction. All patients and controls were given the Holmes and Rahe (1967) Social Readjustment Rating Scale (a scale listing 62 life events that might have been experienced (1) during the six months preceding the onset of depression by patients and (2) the year preceding the interview by the controls (Holmes and Rahe, 1967). The events ranged from death of a spouse to receiving a citation for a traffic violation. The authors divided some of the events into entrance events (such as marriage and birth of a child) and exit events (such as divorce and death of a close family member). There was no significant difference between the patients and controls for entrance events but a fivefold greater likelihood of exit events being reported by the patients than the controls. The author concluded that life stress (especially exit events) is implicated in the causal web of clinical depression.

INTRODUCTION

Most of the chapters in this book present specific methods for determining the association between risk factors and the onset of psychiatric disorders (longitudinal studies, case-control studies, etc.). Other chapters present the statistical methods for assessing the association between putative risk factors and psychiatric disorders. The purpose of these methods is to establish a cause–effect relationship between biological, psychological, and/or social factors and psychiatric disorders.

Yet these methods are based on philosophical and mathematical approaches to "how we know," that is, epistemology. Clinical research attempts to answer questions which will increase our knowledge. How do investigators know they are asking the appropriate and answerable questions? How do they know the methods employed to answer these questions are based upon sound reasoning? How do they know the answers obtained from a study are actually answers to the questions posed? What confidence can be placed in these answers? The research methodologies described are based on philosophical and mathematical approaches to knowing, which include empirical reasoning, inductive logic, laws of probability, and an assumption that the vast majority of psychiatric disorders are caused by multiple factors, i.e., a web of causation. In this chapter the means by which these approaches (in contrast, for example, to deductive logic) assist investigators in gaining confidence that they actually do learn from the studies they perform are described. The hypothesis that stressful life events cause (or contribute to the etiology of) psychiatric disorders will be used to illustrate the philosophy analyzing the methods of patient-oriented research.

Causal inference is the process by which causes are related to the effects they produce. A cause is *necessary* when it always precedes an event. For example, a genetic abnormality is necessary for the onset of Huntington's disease. A cause is *sufficient* when it inevitably initiates or produces an effect. For example, excess alcohol intake inevitably leads to ataxia and slurring of speech though the dose that represents "excess" may vary from one person to another. Causes may be *necessary but not sufficient* in their contribution to a particular outcome. For example, the loss of a loved one is necessary for the diagnosis of bereavement but it is not sufficient. That is, not everyone who loses a loved one experiences bereavement following the loss. An older woman who has been a caretaker for her husband over many years while the husband has suffered from Alzheimer's disease may only experience relief—not bereavement—at the husband's death.

HISTORICAL REVIEW

Two basic but competing approaches to causal inference undergird our thinking about causality. The first is rationalism, which goes back to Plato. According to Plato, knowledge (for our purposes, knowledge about the cause of a psychiatric disorder) is obtained through reason and intuition, not observation. For example, it is intuitive that a person would become depressed if he or she loses his or her job. Clinicians therefore might rationalize that job loss will cause the onset of a depressive episode. In contrast to rationalism, Francis Bacon and others advocated empiricism as the appropriate approach to establishing a causal relationship. In this case, a clinician observes that John Smith becomes depressed following the loss of his job and, based upon many such observations, reasons that depression may follow the loss of a job. There have been many examples of rationalism leading to certain causal explanations of illnesses and their cures that only later were demonstrated to be false or incomplete through empirical studies. For example, Hippocrates rationalized that disease is caused by imbalance of bodily humors (or fluids). Melancholia (severe depression) was believed to derive from an excess of black bile. Relieving the body of black bile through bleeding was thought to relieve melancholia. During the early 19th century, however, bleeding was compared to conservative management of many illnesses. Conservative management was superior to bleeding. Henceforth, bleeding was no longer an acceptable cure for melancholia. Current approaches to establishing causation usually derive from empirical observation as opposed to rationalism.

Closely related to rationalism and empiricism are the concepts of deduction and induction. Aristotle was a proponent of deductive reasoning, i.e., conclusions rationally follow from a premise. For example, Paykel could have begun with the premise that stressful life events cause the onset of clinical depression based upon a theory he conceived in his library. Yet deduction is potentially a closed system. Given the presupposition that stressful events lead to clinical depression, if John experiences a stressful event, then a depressive episode should follow, just as melancholia should follow an excess of black bile. Deductive reason tends to limit the power of unbiased observation. In contrast, induction is a more open system which suggests that conclusions must derive from specific facts. Mary, John, and Jim experience a clinical depression following a stressful life event. Therefore, Paykel might hypothesize that stressful events are a cause of clinical depression after observing many instances of depression following life events.

Observation of specific events by clinicians usually leads to the development of hypotheses which in turn can be tested, i.e., inductive reasoning. Induction as an approach to establishing causal inference, however, cannot establish logical necessity. Conclusive verification of a causal relationship is virtually impossible through empirical, inductive patient-oriented research in psychiatry. Therefore, most hypotheses are tested based on the probability that they are correct—hence, the introduction of mathematical (statistical) approaches. For example, the odds of experiencing an acute life stressor may be five times greater in persons who are clinically depressed compared with persons in the community with a greater than 99% probability that the elevation in risk is true (i.e., $p < .01$). The study of the associations of hypothesized causative agents and psychiatric disorders is limited to estimates of probability; it does not include absolute laws of causality. One might say that the psychiatric investigator thinks more like a gambler than a prophet. Therefore, truth is approached through successive approximations. For example, the Paykel study is one study in a series of studies over time which have progressively established the causation of depression by social stress.

This inductive approach is limited by yet another factor beyond that of probability. Perhaps the philosopher in modern times who was most critical of what we can and cannot demonstrate using empirical, inductive investigative methods was Karl Popper (1965). Popper argued that hypotheses about the empirical world, such as the hypothesis that stressful life events lead to clinical depression, can never be proven by inductive logic. In other words, induction could never prove all current and future associations of stressful events and depression are associated. These hypotheses can only be disproved or "falsified." In patient-oriented research, the hypothesis is worded so that it can be proven false and labeled the *null hypothesis*. In this case the null hypothesis is: "Stressful life events are not associated with clinical depression." It is the "alternate" hypothesis that the investigator actually expects to find, intuitively, i.e., the investigator "intuits" that a life crisis is likely to cause clinical depression. Then, if the investigator observes that persons experiencing depression are more likely to report an acute crisis than persons who do not experience a depression, the null hypothesis is falsified. The investigator has not "proven," however, that stressful life events cause clinical depression. The empirical content of an hypothesis, i.e., the part of the hypothesis which can be observed, is measured by how falsifiable the hypothesis is. For example, the hypothesis that "Stressful life events cause depression" can be placed within an empirical context and tested because it can be falsified, whereas the hypothesis "God is unity" cannot (Rothman, 1986).

The logic of inductive causal reasoning was applied to medicine during the nineteenth century primarily through the work of Koch (1884). He noted that it was not sufficient to establish only the association between a disease and a postulated causative agent: The agent must also be shown to be the "real cause." According to Koch, a causal relationship can be established when:

- The agent is present in every case of the disease.
- The agent is isolated from the diseased host and grown in pure culture.
- The specific disease is reproduced by the agent (in Koch's example) when a pure culture of a microorganism is inoculated into a healthy susceptible host
- The agent is recoverable once again from the experimentally infected host.

Clearly these criteria are neither met by nor applicable to most psychiatric disorders or their etiology. Koch's conditions require that a single cause lead to a single effect, not multiple effects. For most psychiatric disorders a single causative agent, such as a stressful event, can lead to a variety of disorders, such as anxiety disorders, acute psychotic episodes, and depression. In addition, multiple causative agents are necessary to cause a psychiatric disorder. When multiple causative and/or protective factors are involved in the causation of a psychiatric disorder, they may interact in complex ways, in what has been called a "web of causation." Imagine a spider's web: Each strand on the web represents a causative or etiologic factor, and each intersection of strands represents the interaction of these factors. In Chapter 12, methods for analyzing these complex interactions are described. Koch explained the cause of anthrax (anthrax bacillus) using his criteria. For the purposes of this chapter, it is sufficient to recognize that few psychiatric disorders are as simply explained. Stressful events cannot be eliminated as a potential cause of a disorder if there is no specificity. That is, if stressful events lead to the onset of a clinical depression in one person, they may also be the cause of an acute psychosis in another. Furthermore, if clinical depression is caused by a stressful life event, it may also be caused by exposure to a medication such a reserpine.

The factors considered in the causation of disease may be usefully categorized as *predisposing, enabling, precipitating, and reinforcing factors*. In the causal relationship between stressful life events and major depression, a history of major depression is an example of a predisposing factor: a factor which prepares, sensitizes, or otherwise renders the subject more susceptible to the development of the illness. Likewise, individuals who have experienced episodes of depression in the past are more likely to do so in the future. Inadequate social support is an example of an enabling factor, i.e., a factor which facilitates the manifestation of a disease. Stressful life events are less likely to lead to a depressive disorder in persons with adequate social support than in individuals with inadequate social support. The stressful life event itself would be considered a precipitating factor: a factor associated with definitive onset of the disease. The loss of a job which precipitates an episode of major depression would be a specific example of a factor which precipitates a depressive disorder. If a person suffers from a chronic physical illness, this illness might be a *reinforcing factor*: a factor which tends to or aggravate the presence of a depressive disorder. In longitudinal studies, depression is associated with the onset of poor health and poor health is associated with the onset of depressive disorders. Therefore, depressive disorders and poor physical health tend to reinforce one another. Obviously, some factors may be placed into more than one of these categories even for the same episode of illness in an individual. For example, a physical illness may precipitate the onset of a depressive disorder and thereafter the physical illness and depressive disorder reinforce one another.

There are six useful steps that can be taken to establish a cause–effect relationship between a causative agent and a disease. The names of these steps are association, strength of association, biologic credibility, consistency with other investigators, time sequence, and dose–response relationship (Rothman, 1986; Hennekens et al., 1987). The first step in establishing a relationship between a stressful life event and a depressive episode is to identify the association between the stressful event and the disease. The intuitive relationship between stressful events and depressive symptoms has been evident since antiquity. The death of a family member is a good example of such event. For example, King David of Israel, upon hearing that his rebellious son, Absalom, had died, "was shaken. He went up to the room over the gateway and wept" (The Bible, 2 Sam. 18: 33 International Version). Eric Lindemann, in 1945, described a series of depressive symptoms which he labeled "abnormal bereavement" in his subset of 101 subjects who had lost a close relative during the Coconut Grove fire in Boston (Lindemann, 1944). These symptoms included *withdrawal of relationships with others, poor social interaction, self-deprecatory activities*, and *an agitated depression.*

If an association is established, the likelihood of a causal relationship is stronger if the association is strong. The stronger the association, the less likely the relationship is secondary to some other factor which may be confounding the relationship between a putative causal agent, e.g., a stressful event, and an outcome such as depression. For example, Paykel et al. calculated, on the basis of retrospective data, that following the experience of an exit event, the risk for developing a depressive disorder increased fivefold (Paykel et al., 1969). Others have suggested that the increased risk for developing a depressive disorder following a stressful event is about threefold (Bebbington et al., 1992). Most estimates of *relative risk* (see Chapter 3) in epidemiologic studies are of the magnitude of three or less. The sixfold relative risk described by Paykel would be strong evidence for a causative relationship between stressful events and depression, particularly if these data were verified in other studies. In fact, most other studies have not verified such a strength of association as described by Paykel (Bebbington, 1992).

Cause–effect relationship is further strengthened if a biologic mechanism can be proposed to explain the increased risk. The lack of a biological explanation, however, does not undermine the credibility of the statistical association. In fact, a strong association in an epidemiologic study may lead to a search for biological mechanisms. For example, the statistical association found initially between smoking and adenocarcinoma of the lung was not substantiated by a biologic explanation, but many studies since the initial association was established have been directed toward identifying that biological explanation. A number of theories have been suggested to explain the biological mechanism at work in the association between stressful events and depression. For example, it is well known that stress leads to increased production of cortisol, and increased cortisol levels have been associated with major depression (Turpin and Lader, 1984; Selye, 1956; Carroll et al., 1981). Our present knowledge suggests that there are potential psychobiological "causal pathways" relating stressful events to depressive disorders, but none of these has been verified to date. In other words, the cause–effect relationship does have biologic credibility but no proven pathway has been identified.

A fourth step in identifying a relationship between cause and effect is consistency across investigators. Clinical studies, by their very nature, are not as exact as laboratory studies. Consistency across studies, however, provides more confidence in a relationship initially identified in an epidemiologic study. The relationship between stressful events and depression has been verified by many investigators. Though specific differences across studies do emerge (for example, it has been suggested that stressful events are less likely to lead to a depressive disorder in older persons compared to younger persons), most studies have demonstrated the association between stressful events and depression (Paykel, 1979; Fava et al., 1981; Henderson et al., 1981; Bebbington et al., 1992; George et al., 1989).

Perhaps the most critical, or among the most critical, steps in establishing a causal relationship is to document that the exposure of interest precedes the outcome by a period of time consistent with any proposed biologic or psychosocial mechanism. In other words, for stressful events to cause depression, they should precede the onset of the depressive episode. There have been a number of studies which have identified this temporal relationship. For example, Dalgard and colleagues, in a ten-year follow-up survey of 503 persons in Oslo, found that stressful life events predicted depression in this longitudinal study, yet the relationship is "buffered" by a strong supportive network (Dalgard et al., 1966). In most studies which document an association between stressful events and depression, the strength of the association typically is lower in longitudinal compared to cross-sectional studies. This is not unusual in epidemiologic studies.

Finally, to establish a causal relationship, it would be valuable to show a *dose–response* relationship. In other words, if there is a causal relationship between stressful events and depression, then an increased number or severity of stressful events should increase the risk for depression. The greater the stress, the more likely depression will ensue. Numbers of events have been much less studied than severity of events. The risk posed by severity of events has been more often studied than number of events. For example, Brown and colleagues found that the risk of becoming depressed after a severe event is about sixfold during the nine-month period following the event, a very high risk (Brown and Harriss, 1978).

The relationship between social factors, especially psychosocial stress and psychiatric disorders, is a complex one. We have simplified this discussion to illustrate the reasoning used for establishing a causal relationship above. If the reader wishes to explore this issue in more depth, several extensive discussions are listed in the references (Henderson et al., 1981; Turpin and Lader, 1984; Lin et al., 1986).

Problem Set

Gallo et al. (1993) hypothesized that low educational achievement and, separately, unemployment would each increase risk for the onset of depression in middle age and late life. Their prospective study of incident major depression within age and neighborhood subgroups differed from other studies that had examined the prevalence of depression, which were retrospective in their assessments, and which did not account for neighborhood characteristics—such as rate of unemployment, poverty, anomie, and crowding. During one year of follow-up time, the investigators observed 180 new cases of major depression among 7,397 previously unaffected adults aged 40 years and older living in the five metropolitan areas sampled for the NIMH Epidemiologic Catchment Area (ECA) Program: Los Angeles; St. Louis; Baltimore; Durham, NC; and New Haven, CT. Incident cases were compared to 960 noncases from the same census tracts and age strata. Table 1–1 presents the estimated relative risk of major depression associated with low education, unemployment, gender, minority status, and marital status. (The confounding effects of age and census tract were also controlled but not displayed.) Lack of a high school diploma, female gender, nonminority status, and being separated or divorced increased the risk of first onset of a major depressive

TABLE 1–1. Adjusted estimates of relative risk for several major depression risk factors, holding constant all other covariates

SUSPECTED RISK FACTORS IN THE PRIMARY MODEL	RELATIVE RISK ESTIMATE	p VALUE
Low education		
0–11 years of schooling	2.22	<.001
12 years or more	1.00	
Unemployment		
Not working for pay	1.48	.164
Working for pay	1.00	
Sex		
Female	1.77	.006
Male	1.00	
Minority status		
Nonminority	3.84	.001
Minority	1.00	
Marital status		
Separated-divorced	2.03	.012
All other marital	1.00	

From Gallo et al., 1993

TABLE 1–2. Estimates of relative risk for major depression, modeled with an interaction of educational attainment and gender, holding constant baseline employment, minority, and marital status

	RELATIVE RISK ESTIMATE	95% CONFIDENCE INTERVAL
Women with 0–11 years of schooling	3.26	(1.78, 5.95)
Women with 12+ years of schooling	1.12	(.63, 1.99)
Men with 0–11 years of schooling	1.21	(.60, 2.46)
Men with 12+ years of schooling	1.00	

episode (MDE). Table 1–2 displays the relative risk for first-onset MDE associated with both being female and lacking a high school diploma. Elevated risk associated with low education was specific to women only.

Questions

1. If lack of a high school diploma were a sufficient cause of unremitting major depression, (a) what variable would provide all necessary information regarding the cause of single-onset MDE, and (b) what prescribed treatment would be standard for all patients with MDE? If lack of a high school diploma were a necessary but not a sufficient cause, how would this differ?

2. What is the benefit of examining a broad array of risk factors for first onset of major depression?

3. In Table 1–1, which of the significant risk factors for first onset MDE might be categorized as predisposing, enabling, precipitating, or reinforcing factors?

4. Using Tables 1–1 and 1–2, evaluate the six types of evidence typically used to establish a cause–effect relationship—in this case, between low educational achievement and incident major depression.

Answers

1. If lack of a high school diploma were a sufficient cause of a MDE, the assessment of educational achievement would be sufficient to determine the risk of major depression, and a high school remediation program would be standard and effective treatment. If low educational achievement were a necessary but not a sufficient cause of major depression, then all individuals experiencing MDE would report lack of a high school diploma, but other risk factors would distinguish such undereducated MDE patients from persons without a high school diploma who did not experience MDE.

2. Risk of a chronic psychiatric disorder such as major depression is embedded in a complex interaction of genetic, clinical, and environmental factors. Without

controlling for the effects of multiple risk factors that may themselves be over-
lapping or interactive, it is not possible to identify those risk factors which are direct and those which work indirectly through other risk factors or are potentiated
by other risk factors. For example, the evidence is inconsistent regarding the risk
of depression associated with educational underachievement. In particular, that relationship may be confounded by poor physical health, deficient social support, or
the lack of access to material rewards associated with education, such as health
care (Harlow et al., 1991; Kennedy et al., 1989; Phifer and Murrell, 1986).

3. Gender and race might be considered predisposing factors because they are
established at birth. Likewise, education is an early antecedent variable which may
predispose individuals to an episode of major depression in late life. Marital status may operate as either an enabling or precipitating factor. If being separated or
divorced is a "chronic" situation, it may enable the development of depressive
symptoms. On the other hand, if the event of becoming separated or divorced occurred between *time 1* and *time 2* assessments, one might speculate that the event
itself was a precipitating factor with respect to the depressive episode.

4. The results presented in the tables demonstrated a very strong, statistically
significant association between low educational achievement and incident depression among women, with a marked elevation in risk of more than threefold in this
subgroup. The Gallo et al. paper did not address biologic mechanisms per se, but
it is not implausible to consider the long-standing deficits in health, functional capacity, and health care coverage among less-educated women to be progenitors of
chronic physiologic stress, long implicated in the causal web of mood deficits. The
Gallo et al. results are consonant with multiple U.S. and international studies that
demonstrate a link between education and depression, including Aro et al. (1995)
(Finland), Carpiniello et al. (1989) (Italy), Vazquez-Barquero et al. (1992) (Spain),
Dohrenwend et al. (1992) (Israel), and Blazer et al. (1988) (Durham, NC, USA).
The time sequence of early (usually prior to age 20) educational achievement and
mood disorders in middle or late life is appropriate to a conclusion of causation.
In addition, the measurement of education preceded the onset of the MDE. The
sixth condition, evidence of dose–response, was not addressed in this study inso-
far as educational achievement was dichotomized at 0–11 vs. 12+ years of formal
schooling.

REFERENCES

Aro S., Aro H., Salinto M., Keskimaki I. 1995. Educational level and hospital use in men-
    tal disorders: a population-based study. *Acta Psychiatrica Scandinavica* 91: 305–312.
Bebbington P.E., Stuart E., Tennant C. 1992. Misfortune and resilience: a community study
    of women. *Psychological Medicine* 14: 347–354.
Blazer D., Swartz M., Woodbury M., Manton K.D., Hughes D., George L.K. 1988. De-

pressive symptoms and depressive diagnoses in a community population: use of a new procedure for analysis of psychiatric classification. *Archives of General Psychiatry* 43: 667–675.

Brown G.W., Harriss J.O. Social Origins of Depression. London, Tavistock, 1978.

Carpinello B., Carta M.G., Rudas N. 1989. Depression among elderly people. *Acta Psychiatrica Scandinavia* 80: 445–450.

Carroll B.J., Feinberg M., Graden J.E., Terika J., Albalar F., Haskett R.F., James N.M., Kronfo P.Z., Lohr N., Steiner M., De Vigne J.P., Young E. 1981. A specific laboratory test for the diagnosis of melancholia. Standardization, validation, and clinical utility. *Archives of General Psychiatry* 38: 15–22.

Dalgard O.S., Bjork S., Tambs K. 1966. Social support, negative life events and mental health. *British Journal of Psychiatry* 166: 29–34.

Dohrenwend B.P., Levav I., Shrout P.E., Schwarz S., Naveh G., Link B.G., Skokdon A.E., Stueve A. 1992. Socioeconomic status and psychiatric disorders: the causation-selection issue. *Science* 255: 946–952.

Fava G.A., Munieri F., Pavin L., Kellner R. 1981. Life events and depression: a replication. *Journal of Affective Disorders*. 3: 159–165.

Gallo J.J., Royall D.R., Anthony J.C. 1993. Risk factors for the onset of depression in middle age and later life. *Social Psychiatry and Psychiatric Epidemiology* 28: 101–108.

George L.K., Blazer D.G., Hughes D.C., Fowler N. 1989. Social support in the outcome of major depression. *British Journal of Psychiatry* 154: 478–485.

Harlow S.D., Goldberg E.L., Comstock G.W. 1991. A longitudinal study of risk factors for depressive symptomatology in elderly widows and married women. *American Journal of Epidemiology* 134: 526–538.

Henderson A.S., Byrne D.G., Duncan-Jones P. 1981. *Neurosis and the Social Environment.* Sydney: Academic Press.

Hennekens C.H., Buring J.E., Mayrent S.L. 1987. *Epidemiology in Medicine.* Boston: Little, Brown.

Holmes T.H., Rahe R.H. 1967. The social readjustment rating scale. *Journal of Psychosomatic Research* 11: 213–218.

Kennedy G.J., Kelman H.R., Thomas C., Wisniewski W., Metz H., Bijur P.E. 1989. Hierarchy of characteristics associated with depressive symptoms in an urban elderly sample. *American Journal of Psychiatry* 146: 220–225.

Koch R. 1884. Die aetiologie der Tuberculose. Mitteilungen aus dem Kaiserlichen Gesundheitsamte 2:1.

Lin N., Dean A., Essel W. (eds). 1986. *Social Support: Life Events and Depression.* New York: Academic Press.

Lindemann E. 1944. Symptomatology in management of acute grief. *American Journal of Psychiatry.* 101: 141–149.

Paykel E.S., Meyers J.K., Dienelt M.N., Klerman G.L., Lindenthal J.J., Pepper M.P. 1969. Life events and depression: a controlled study. *Archives of General Psychiatry* 21: 753–760.

Paykel E.S. 1979. Recent life events in the development of the depressive disorders. In *The Psychobiology of Depressive Disorders: Implications for the Effects of Stress* (ed. Depue R.A.), New York: Academic Press.

Phifer J.F., Murrell S. A. 1986. Etiologic factors in the onset of depressive symptoms in older adults. *Journal of Abnormal Psychiatry* 95: 282–291.

Popper K.R. 1965. *The Logic of Scientific Discovery.* New York: Harper & Row.

Rothman K.J. 1986. *Modern Epidemiology.* Boston: Little, Brown.

Selye H. 1956. *The Stress of Life*. New York: McGraw-Hill.

Turpin G., Lader M. 1984. Life events and mental disorders: biological theories of their mode of action. In *Life Events and Psychiatric Disorders: Controversial Issues* (ed. Katschnig H), New York: Cambridge University Press.

Vazquez-Barquero J.L., Manrique J.F.D., Munoz J., Arango J.M., Gaite L., Herrera S., Der, G.J. 1992. Sex differences in mental illness: a community study of the influence of physical health and socio-demographic factors. *Social Psychiatry and Psychiatric Epidemiology* 27: 62–68.

2

REVIEWING A PUBLISHED STUDY

OBJECTIVES

- To describe and critique a published clinical research study.
- To recognize deficits and/or lack of clarity in the background information provided to the reader of a clinical research study.
- To identify the type of study design used in a published study and determine how the investigators attempted to overcome inherent weaknesses of the design.
- To review the study results and draw one's own conclusions from them.
- To critique the conclusions drawn by the authors of a research study in light of their research design and results.

INTRODUCTION

In this chapter we provide guidelines for studying a study. We explain how a critical reader reviews the components of a research report.

The introduction/objectives of the study provide its rationale. The methods section describes the study design, including selection of subjects; identification of independent, dependent, and control variables; the methods of obtaining data from subjects to measure these variables; and the statistical methods for analyzing the data. The results section presents key findings with emphasis on the actual data. In the conclusions section, the authors suggest potential applications of the findings, problems in the study design, and directions for future studies.

No one reads every scientific article critically. We must trust the editors of journals and the reviewers of articles submitted to journals to critique the studies thoroughly before we read them. Therefore, many clinicians scan a journal article simply by reading the abstract and perhaps the introduction/objectives, glancing at one or two tables, and quickly reviewing the conclusions. The abstract is written so that the reader can easily grasp the gist of an article. Readers may thus read the text of the article only to fill in details in which they have an interest. This is appropriate since a critical review of every article in a journal would be an extremely laborious and usually unnecessary task.

Nevertheless, an issue of a journal may contain one or two articles in which the authors address a topic that catches the reader's interest or is relevant to the reader's specific work. These articles are usually read more thoroughly and critically. Perhaps the conclusions are startling or unexpected. Perhaps the reader disagrees with the findings. In addition, many clinicians are asked to review an article being considered for publication in a journal. This is a most important responsibility, for reviewers are the persons who primarily decide whether an article is published or not published.

To protect journal readers, the reviewer must read the article critically and identify flaws. The manuscripts submitted to journals are frequently flawed (would you expect otherwise?), and investigators almost always must revise an article before it is published. In addition, the reviewer has a responsibility to the investigator, for many hours have been put into a study before the article is written. So the reviewer should try to help the investigators present their results more effectively or to draw more realistic conclusions. (Unfortunately, a flawed methodology cannot be corrected in retrospect.) For these reasons, clinicians reading a clinical research report should be able to review the report critically. Guidelines for reviewing a report are presented below and are illustrated by a recent article published in the *Archives of General Psychiatry*. To review a study, the reader must call on his or her clinical knowledge as well as the knowledge of research design described in this book. The review is necessarily time-limited, so a focused approach is necessary. These guidelines are not comprehensive but rather are suggested as a means for cutting to the heart of the study. They are also applicable to "review articles" which critically review the extant literature on a particular topic for a scientific journal. Each article discussed in such a review should be critically evaluated before an appropriate conclusion is drawn from the literature. One additional technique for performing a literature review is "meta-analysis," which is beyond the scope of this book.

A quick review of the major journals in psychiatry, such as the *American Jour-*

nal of Psychiatry, Archives of General Psychiatry, the *British Journal of Psychiatry*, and the *Journal of Affective Disorders* reveals a consistency in the structure of an original report of a person-oriented research study.

ABSTRACT

In recent years, the components of a typical research report have been highlighted in the abstract of the report. For example, a typical abstract in the *American Journal of Psychiatry* includes the objective of the study, the methods, the results, and the conclusions. The *Archives of General Psychiatry* provides, at times, a more detailed abstract which includes objectives, research design, patients, outcome measures, results, and conclusions.

The abstract should contain, at a glance, the research questions, rationale, study design, conclusions (with some data) and implications of the study for the reader. Abstracts are limited, usually to fewer than 200 words, so economy in providing this information is central to the task of preparing the abstract. Other than clarity constrained by economy, the most frequent problem found with abstracts is that they are at some variance with the actual article. That is, a reviewer may critique the abstract as misrepresenting the study findings.

BACKGROUND AND OBJECTIVES

When reading the background and objectives of an article (usually contained in the introduction to the article), the reader should be able to identify what the authors intend to learn from a study and why that study will contribute to the understanding of a psychiatric disorder and its treatment. The following questions should be answered:

- What are the objectives and specific aims of the study? Do the authors state their objectives and aims clearly and concisely? (See Chapter 1.)
- Do the authors provide a rationale for the objectives of the study? In other words, is this a study worth doing?
- What prior research will the study build upon?
- What is not known that will be made known by the study?
- Do the authors propose explicit hypotheses? (Chapter 1.) That is, have they made an educated guess as to what they expect to find at the conclusion of the study?

A review of a recent article by Paul H. Soloff and colleagues provides an opportunity to illustrate the critique of a study. The authors describe a randomized clinical trial designed to compare the efficiency of the neuroleptic haloperidol with the monoamine oxidase inhibitor antidepressant phenelzine sulfate in treating specific symptoms of patients with borderline personality disorder. If haloperidol proved more effective in treating symptoms such as impulsive-aggressive behavior and phenelzine was more effective in treating symptoms such as despair, then response to medication could provide a means for defining subcategories of borderline personality disorder, i.e., affective and schizotypal subtypes.

What Are the Overall Objectives and Specific Aims of the Study?

The authors clearly state their objectives in the introduction to the article: "to compare the efficacy of a neuroleptic (haloperidol) to a monoamine oxidase inhibitor antidepressant (phenelzine sulfate) against the . . . symptoms of . . . borderline inpatients in an effort to dissect affective and schizotypal symptom patterns of subgroups using medication response."

In the introduction, however, the authors do not describe what they are actually going to do in order to accomplish these objectives. (In the methods section, the authors describe a randomized, double-blind, placebo-controlled trial [see Chapter 9].) It would be helpful for the authors to describe briefly the study population and design in the introduction prior to the detailed description of the methods later in paper.

Do the Authors Provide a Rationale for the Objectives of this Study?

The authors inform us that "Borderline personality disorder (BPD) is a heterogeneous syndrome manifested by a vulnerability to affective instability, cognitive-perceptual distortions, and behavioral discontrol in the context of a chronically unstable interpersonal style." Patients therefore present with varying symptom pictures, and current diagnostic categories alone do not always permit disaggregating the subtypes of BPD. From their own work and the work of other investigators, neuroleptic medications have been reported efficacious against a "broad spectrum of symptoms of patients with borderline personality disorder, including depression, anger and hostility, impulsiveness, and especially against schizotypal features, such as paranoid ideation, illusions and ideas of reference." Antidepressant medications, both tricyclic antidepressants and selective serotonin reuptake inhibitors, have been somewhat efficacious in treating symptoms such as depression, hostility, obsessive-compulsive symptoms, and impulsivity. Monoamine oxidase inhibitors have been reported efficacious against depressed mood and behavioral impulsivity. The authors therefore provide evidence that different medications may be effective against different types of symptoms in BPD patients; therefore, perhaps medication response will help differentiate these patients. They do not inform the reader, however, why they selected a monoamine oxidase inhibitor as opposed to a tricyclic antidepressant or a selective serotonin reuptake inhibitor. In summary, there appears to be a rationale for the study of subtyping BPD based on response to different kinds of medications but the rationale is less clear for the specific selection of medications. To their credit, there was no previous literature to guide them in their selection.

What Was Not Known That Will Be Made Known From the Study?

The authors inform the reader that "pharmacologic dissection of an affective borderline subtype using antidepressant medication has not been successfully demonstrated." Therefore, this study should help determine whether pharmacologic response can be useful in differentiating an affective subtype of borderline personality disorder which responds to antidepressant medications.

Do the Authors Propose Explicit Hypotheses?

The authors do not propose explicit hypotheses. However, the authors suggest a distinct possibility of finding an affective and a schizotypal subtype of BPD which can be identified through pharmacologic response to an antidepressant or neuroleptic medication. The implied null hypothesis (see Chapter 1) is, "There will be no subtypes of BPD based on response to antidepressants and neuroleptic medications."

METHODS

Many clinicians do not read the Methods of a study in detail. They don't have the time. The *American Journal of Psychiatry* and the *Archives of General Psychiatry* both provide a brief description of the methods in the abstract (and this is generally sufficient to gain some understanding of the design of the study). Clinicians who shape their practices based on findings from the literature, however, should develop the ability to critique the methods of a study. Many methodological flaws ultimately derive from a lack of *clinical* understanding of the behavior of diseases in populations and their response to treatment. The following questions should be asked regarding the methods:

- What is the study design (descriptive study, cohort study, case-control study, clinical trial)? (See Chapters 5, 7, 8, 9.)
- How are the subjects selected? (See Chapter 9.)
- Is there an appropriate control group? (See Chapter 3.)
- Are there enough subjects to test the hypotheses? (See Chapter 12.)
- What are the independent, dependent, and control variables? (See Chapter 3.)

- How are they measured? (See Chapter 3.)
- What are the potential biases in the study? (See Chapter 9.)
- Was human subject approval obtained? If so, how?

What Is the Study Design?

In the article by Soloff and colleagues, the study design was a randomized, double-blind, placebo-controlled trial (see Chapter 9). One hundred eight consecutively admitted BPD patients were randomly assigned, initially, to treatment with phenelzine ($n = 38$), haloperidol ($n = 36$), and placebo ($n = 34$). All subjects were free of medication for 7 days prior to the onset of the study. Doses of medication were titrated up to 4 mg of haloperidol q.d. or 60 mg of phenelzine sulfate q.d. or four tablets of placebo q.d. within 1 week. A second week allowed for adjustment and stabilization of the dose. All patients who entered the study remained in the hospital for a minimum of 2 weeks once begun on medication, and then patients were followed for 5 weeks of acute treatment followed by 16 weeks of continuation of treatment for medication responders.

This design is typical of a randomized, double-blind placebo-controlled study (though the reader is not told by what means the patients were randomized) (see Chapter 9). The actual study continued for the 5 weeks, following the initial 2 weeks of the study. See Figure 2–1 for a diagram of the study design.

How Were the Subjects Selected?

In this study, patients were recruited from the inpatient services of the Western Psychiatric Institute and Clinic of the University of Pittsburgh School of Medicine. Patients were included if they received a diagnosis of BPD and if they scored 7 or greater on the Diagnostic Interview for Borderline Patients (Gunderson et al., 1981). The Schedule for Affective Disorders and Schizophrenia (SADS) was used to determine comorbidity, and patients were excluded if they suffered from a current or lifetime diagnosis of schizophrenia, schizoaffective disorder, manic disorder, bipolar disorder with mania or hypomania, or psychotic major depression. In addition, patients were excluded if they exhibited evidence of drug and/or alcohol-related deficits or physical dependency, central nervous system disease (including recent electroconvulsive therapy), physical disorders of known psychiatric consequence, or borderline mental retardation. The subjects therefore went through an extensive screening process in order that the investigators could study BPD uncontaminated by other serious psychiatric disorders.

The investigators do not inform the reader about the type of patients admitted to the Western Psychiatric Institute and Clinic (and therefore the reader cannot assess the population from which this sample is drawn). In fact, the Western Psychiatric Institute admits a heterogeneous group of patients. Inclusion and exclu-

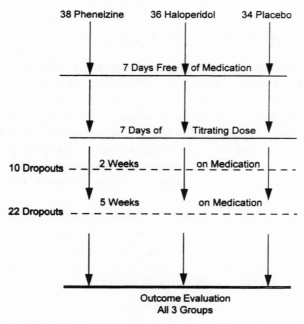

Clinical Trials
Inpatient Services of
Western Psychiatric Clinics

108 Subjects with Borderline Personality Disorder
(Random Assignment into 3 Groups)

38 Phenelzine   36 Haloperidol   34 Placebo

7 Days Free of Medication

7 Days of Titrating Dose

10 Dropouts — — 2 Weeks — — — on Medication — — —

5 Weeks   on Medication
22 Dropouts — — — — — — — — — — — — —

Outcome Evaluation
All 3 Groups

FIGURE 2–1. Diagram of a study design of the study by Soloff et al. (1993).

sion criteria were explicitly stated. Therefore, these investigators provide us with enough information so the reader can feel reasonably comfortable in assuming that the subjects do represent the general population of BPD patients not comorbid with other serious psychotic disorders.

These investigators do not inform us, however, as to how many subjects were omitted from the study due to the exclusion criteria. If this information were available to us, the reader could better evaluate in what ways the subjects studied vary from patients with features of BPD typically evaluated and treated on inpatient psychiatric services.

All of these study patients were admitted to the hospital. Did this have any adverse affect on selection? Some patients who met criteria for inclusion in the study probably did not agree to be admitted to the hospital. Other patients may have been so severely ill that they were eliminated from the 108 subjects who eventually participated in the study.

Is There an Appropriate Control Group?

In a randomized, double-blind, placebo-controlled trial, neither patients nor persons rating the patients in such a study know what medication the patient is receiving. Approximately one-third of the patients received a placebo, and the group receiving placebo was randomly selected. Therefore, an appropriate control group was available for comparison with the two experimental groups.

Are There Enough Subjects to Test the Hypothesis?

To determine the number of subjects necessary to test the hypothesis, one should perform a power analysis (see Chapter 9). This power analysis, however, assumes that the investigator has some estimate of the effect which she or he expects to find if the hypothesis is to be verified (or disproved). For example, the investigator studying whether a new antihypertensive agent is effective in lowering blood pressure should estimate how much a new agent might be expected to lower blood pressure compared to a standard treatment (such as hydrochlorothiazide). Then simple formulas are available to identify the number of subjects needed to test the hypothesis.

Unfortunately, in many psychiatric investigations, investigators have no idea what degree of effect to expect. In this study the investigators probably had no guidelines. The study is a relatively large clinical trial. Yet we have no way of knowing whether the number of subjects available in this study was sufficient in order to determine if different subtypes can be distinguished.

What Are the Predictor, Outcome, Dependent, and Control Variables? How Are They Measured?

The predictor or independent variables in this study were the medications used (phenelzine and haloperidol). The outcome or dependent variables were depression, global symptom severity, anxiety, anger-hostility, and psychoticism/impulsivity. Depression was measured by frequently used scales, including the Hamilton Depression Scale (two versions), the Beck Depression Inventory, the depression scale of the Symptom Check List (SCL)-90, and an Inventory of Atypical Depression (including reactivity, hypersomnia, increased appetite, weight gain, and rejection sensitivity). Global symptom severity was measured by the Global Assessment Scale (GAS) and the SCL-90 global symptom index. Anxiety was measured by the anxiety scale of the SCL-90 and the obsessive-compulsive scale of the SCL-90. Anger-hostility was measured by the hostility scale of the SCL-90 and the IMPS Hostility Scale. Psychoticism was measured by the Schizotypal Symptoms Index, the SCL-90 paranoid scale, and the SCL-90 psychoticism scale. Impulsivity was measured by the Ward Scale of Impulse Action, the Barratt Impulsiveness Scale, and the Self-Report of Impulse Control. Other than grouping these assessment procedures together, the authors basically reported each scale result before and after treatment for the three treatment groups (phenelzine sulfate, haloperidol, and placebo) and compared these using both t-tests and analysis of covariance (see Chapter 12). Baseline depression was controlled by analysis of covariance in this study, but otherwise there were no control variables (see Chapter 3). In other words, the investigators simply compared before and after scores on the different scales used in the study.

Though this is a relatively large clinical study, the investigators may be faulted for using too many assessment scales before and after treatment. In fact, they used 24 different measures in their initial comparisons and 16 different measures in the analysis of covariance. This presents potential problems, for statistically significant associations between the variables measured could arise by chance (see Chapter 12). The use of too many scales also reflects a lack of specificity either in defining the dependent major variables or in measuring a specific dependent variable. For example, the study would have been more specific if the investigators had measured the dependent variable depression with one scale only.

What Are the Potential Biases in the Study?

Two causes of potential bias in this study have already been mentioned. First, we do not know from what population the final sample was selected (and what factors contributed to subjects not participating in the study). Therefore, the group of BPD patients studied by these investigators may not represent the clinical population of BPD patients. Perhaps they do, but not enough information is provided to be certain. The second potential bias is the number of measures used for the dependent variables of interest. The tactics used by these investigators are unfortunately typical of investigators in pharmacologic trials. Specifically, they use multiple measures across multiple domains of interest but provide little rationale for the selection of the measures. In other words, this study is made more confusing by the lack of specificity in defining and measuring the dependent variables.

Was Human Subject Approval Obtained? If So, How?

Many journals now insist that reports which involve experimental investigation (such as obtaining blood samples from subjects) and interviews of subjects must include a statement that written informed consent was obtained after the procedures were fully explained. The journals rely upon the institutions from which the investigators derive to ensure "full explanation." Specifically, institutions where research is performed upon human subjects appoint an Institutional Review Board (IRB), which includes not only basic science and clinical science investigators but also representatives of the public, ethicists, and persons with legal expertise. The process of obtaining IRB approval is more detailed today than in the past and may take 4 to 6 weeks for completion.

Related to IRB approval is a statement of authorship and full disclosure. For an author to be included on an accepted manuscript, there must be evidence that sufficient effort was made to ensure that she/he can vouch for the amassing of data presented and the integrity of the scientific information reported.

Full disclosure necessitates that the author(s) assure the journal that the data and discussion submitted have not been previously published, i.e., that the contribution is original. In addition, the author(s) must reveal financial arrangements (such as stock held in a pharmaceutical company or support of the research by a pharmaceutical company) that might bias the report of results. Other potential sources of bias (such as a vested interest in the results) should also be disclosed.

In the report of the Soloff et al. study, the authors indicate that informed consent was obtained. They also note that the research was supported by the National Institute of Mental Health (no support from pharmaceutical companies), so it appears that the authors have met the standards for both informed consent and full disclosure.

RESULTS

Presentation of the results of a research report is the heart of the report. Readers too often, however, jump to the conclusions and discussion sections without carefully analyzing the results of the study. The following questions should be asked regarding the results:

- Do the authors present data in such a way that the reader can independently interpret the data?
- Are tables and figures used effectively to display the results?
- Are tables and figures used without bias in the display of results?
- Do the authors summarize accurately in the text the data presented in tables and figures?
- What statistical tests are used to demonstrate statistical significance? Are the tests appropriate to the data? (See Chapter 12.)

In the study reported by Soloff and colleagues, the results were presented in both the text of the paper and in two tables.

Do the Authors Present Data in Such a Way That the Reader Can Independently Interpret the Data?

In the first table of their paper, the authors presented before and after scores for each of the measures of depression, anxiety, anger-hostility/psychoticism, and impulsivity, which permits an easy review by the reader of the results. Their data for two measures are abstracted in Table 2–1.

TABLE 2–1. Psychological measures before versus after treatment[a] $\overline{\chi}$ (SD)

PSYCHOLOGICAL MEASURES	PHENELZINE SULFATE (n = 34)		HALOPERIDOL (n = 30)		PLACEBO (n = 28)	
	BEFORE	AFTER	BEFORE	AFTER	BEFORE	AFTER
Depression: Ham-D-24	24.35(6.38)	13.50(7.71)	25.83(4.68)	18.60(7.44)	25.79(6.79)	15.04(9.02)
Psychoticism: SCL-90/Paranoid	1.84(.92)	0.92(.87)	1.89(1.04)	1.06(.96)	2.03(.92)	1.18(.98)

[a] p < .001, two-tailed t-test

From Soloff et al., 1993

Specifically, they presented the mean and standard deviation (variation from the mean) for the three groups before and after treatment. They use, in each case, a t-test (see Chapter 12) to determine if the differences for each group before and after treatment are statistically significant.

In a second table they compare the three groups using analysis of covariance (ANCOVA) to determine if the groups differ in results when both two-way and three-way comparisons are made. An excerpt of this table is presented in Table 2–2 for two measures.

This table presents the key, for the authors are attempting to differentiate subtypes of borderline personality by response to medication. These data provide virtually everything we need to critique their results. As can be seen, the medications do not appear to differentiate subtypes: One medication does not appear to be consistently superior to another across the different domains explored. Overall results are similar to the abstract of the two measures presented in Table 2–2.

The authors also provide important data for analyzing any clinical trial in the text—data regarding attrition or drop-out from the study. There were 32 dropouts from the study, 10 of whom dropped out before 2 weeks of medications and 22 of whom dropped out after 2 or more weeks but less than 5 weeks of medication. They also analyzed the dropouts to determine if there were significant differences in attrition across the medication groups and did not find a difference.

Are Tables and Figures Used Effectively and Without Bias?

The first table is "busy," given that the authors present results from multiple symptom scales, yet useful for someone studying this article in depth. The full table contains approximately 180 numbers, including means and standard deviations. The second table is even more complex. First, the authors present a three-way analysis of covariance of the effectiveness of haloperidol vs. phenelzine sulfate vs. placebo for 16 different measures. If one understands analysis of covariance, one quickly recognizes that this column simply indicates whether the therapies were significantly different across the different domains explored, such as depression, psychoticism, impulsivity, and anxiety. According to the significance tests, there was virtually no difference in effectiveness. The remaining three columns are more easy to interpret. Specifically, two-way comparisons are presented for medications (placebo vs. haloperidol, placebo vs. phenelzine, and haloperidol vs. phenelzine) across these same domains. Again, no significant differences were consistently found when comparing therapies across domains. A slight trend did appear in favor of phenelzine as a more effective therapy for depressive symptoms and haloperidol as more effective for hostility and impulsivity. Neither table contains significant bias. What is less clear from the tables, however, is the overall effectiveness of these medications for improving symptoms. For the most part, in Table 2–1, before-treatment symptoms are more severe than after-treatment symptoms,

TABLE 2–2. Between-group comparisons after treatment[a]

| | THREE-WAY | PAIRWISE | | |
		HALOPERIDOL VS.	PHENELZINE VS.	HALOPERIDOL VS.
	Haloperidol vs. Phenelzine vs. Placebo	Placebo	Placebo	Phenelzine
Depression (Ham-D-17)	NS	NS	NS	4.06 (<.05)[b]
Psychoticism (SCL-90/Paranoid)	NS	NS	NS	3.04 (<.1)[b]

[a]ANCOVA indicates analysis of covariance with baseline as covariate. Values are F-test results with the p value in parentheses

[b]Phenelzine > haloperidol

From Soloff et al., 1993

even for the placebo treatment. Therefore the lack of difference between drugs may be explained in part by a lack of overall difference between either drug and placebo: Medications are not that effective in treating BPD.

Are the Results Meaningful as Well as Significant?

This study is a "negative study" in that the results refute the hypothesis that pharmacologic response can assist in dissecting the heterogeneity of symptoms in BPD. The lack of significant findings across a wide variety of symptom scales in this study provides a meaningful finding for us: One cannot easily distinguish subtypes of borderline personality disorder by medication response alone. Regarding response to medications, though, some results are statistically significant: phenelzine was significantly better at the 0.05 level in improving scores on the global assessment scale than haloperidol. It is questionable, however, whether these are meaningful results for the difference in the decrease in symptoms was minimal.

What Statistical Tests Are Used to Demonstrate Significance?

Initially, a paired t-test for changes in mean scores for one group over time was used to determine for each treatment group (phenelzine sulfate, haloperidol, placebo) whether symptoms improved over time. This is an appropriate statistical test for comparing changes in continuous variables (such as a symptom scale) from one time to another (see Chapter 12). To perform between-group differences (the principal question addressed in this study), an analysis of covariance was instituted. Analysis of covariance is an appropriate test when the dependent variable is the post-test score (e.g., Ham-D-24), the independent variable is the pretest score and one is comparing two or three groups (see Chapter 12).

CONCLUSIONS AND IMPLICATIONS

The conclusions and implications of a study should derive directly from the methods and results. If the reader is to critique the conclusions, however, or to search for additional conclusions not reported by the authors, the methods and results must be reviewed carefully. A critical review of the conclusions should ask the following questions:

- What are the conclusions drawn by the authors?
- Are the conclusions justified by the results?
- What are the implications?
- Do the authors recognize potential problems with the study design? (See Chapter 9.)

- Do the authors suggest further studies to remedy problems in the present study?

What Are the Conclusions Drawn by the Authors?

Soloff and colleagues concluded that the responses to both medications were not significantly different than placebo, and the responses to medications were modest at best. For example, they noted that though depression scores improved 43.5%, they still fell within the impaired range following treatment. Though overall functioning on Global Assessment improved 33.6%, it still fell in the mildly-to-moderately-impaired range at the end of the 5-week trial. They also failed to demonstrate the efficacy for low-dose neuroleptics over placebo on a broad spectrum of affective, schizotypical, and behavioral symptoms. In addition, they concluded that phenelzine was not an effective treatment for depression in borderline personality disorder. They proposed that the failure of both of these treatments may have been due to the time in hospital before treatment and to in-hospital milieu during treatment. Specifically, time and milieu treatment reduced symptom severity in and of themselves (the placebo group responded as well as the drug groups) but a residual of symptoms remained, especially depressive symptoms, which were refractory to pharmacotherapy.

The authors also concluded appropriately that the strategy of pharmacologic dissection of patients with BPD into categorical subtypes was not productive. Neither phenelzine nor haloperidol proved consistently superior in treating specific domains of interest to the authors: depressions, psychoticisms, anxiety, anger/hostility, and overall function.

Are the Conclusions Justified by the Results?

The authors have taken a conservative approach as they draw conclusions from their data. They recognize the lack of difference between placebo and treatment groups and the inability of pharmacotherapy to discriminate different subtypes of borderline personality disorder. They warn the reader, however, that this study was limited to an inpatient setting and to a relatively short period of evaluation. They caution the reader not to generalize these conclusions to the outpatient setting and suggest that a trial in outpatient settings would complement the current study. The reader can easily accept the conclusions drawn by the authors from the results of their study.

What Are the Implications?

The implications of these findings, according to the authors, were as follows. First, they suggested that the effectiveness of treating the acute symptoms of patients with BPD with pharmacotherapy in inpatient settings was difficult to evaluate because of the powerful and nonspecific response to time and milieu alone, i.e., the placebo effects. Therefore, the relief of acute symptoms associated with hospitalization may have masked the beneficial changes in more chronic symptoms of BPD which may be more responsive to treatment in outpatient settings.

The authors also implied that failure of pharmacologic dissection challenges the basic assumption that the affective, cognitive, and impulsive symptom domains of BPD represent discrete, biologically based trait vulnerabilities and are rather core aspects of the borderline psychopathological condition which are not easily disaggregated. The reader can reasonably accept the implications drawn by the authors.

Do the Authors Admit Potential Problems With Study Design?

The authors of this study were careful to remind the reader of potential methodologic problems. As noted above, a major potential bias was the limitation of the study to an inpatient setting and a relatively short period of follow-up. The authors also raised concerns regarding the characteristics of the subjects in this sample. Specifically, in a retrospective comparison of the patients sampled from this study and a previous study by these investigators, they found that symptom severity among subjects diagnosed with borderline personality disorder in the previous study was significantly greater than in the current study. Therefore, subjects in the present study may have had "less room to improve" during the period of treatment. In addition, more severe symptom presentations in patients have been demonstrated to be more responsive to pharmacologic intervention in previous studies.

They also pointed out that bias may have been introduced by a disproportionate number of subjects with comorbid major depressive disorder and significant depressive symptoms in the haloperidol treatment group at baseline. They suggested that though these subjects were selected randomly, the random selection "stacked the deck" against haloperidol as an effective therapy, for it was to be of little value in treating depression, a frequent symptom in BPD.

Do the Authors Suggest Future Studies to Remedy Problems in the Present Study?

Yes, the authors recommended two additional studies. First, they recommend replicating this study in an outpatient compared to an inpatient setting (a study which they had undertaken). They noted, however, that compliance in a 22-week follow-up study where patients were encouraged to leave the hospital as soon as possible was low: Patients were intolerant of neuroleptic side effects, which added to poorer ratings on symptom scales and increased dropout rates. In other words, the authors recognized that there are no perfect studies and that the best approximation of the efficacy of these medications in treating BPD must derive from multiple studies of both inpatients and outpatients.

No study design or execution is perfect. Despite the problems with this study (a clinician experienced in treating BPD would expect problems in such a study), the editors of the *Archives* decided to publish the results. This paper advances our knowledge and provides us with guidelines for additional studies. Given the state of the art of clinical trials with BPD patients, this was a most reasonable and appropriate strategy to determine if subtypes of BPD could be distinguished via pharmacotherapy.

Problem Set

In 1986, William Summers and colleagues published an article in the *New England Journal of Medicine* describing a clinical trial utilizing tetrahydroaminoacridine (THA) to treat senile dementia of the Alzheimer's type (Summers et al., 1986).[1] In this double-blind crossover study of 17 subjects, the authors found that THA was superior to placebo in improving a number of measures of cognitive performance, suggesting that THA may be one of the effective treatments for Alzheimer's disease.[2]

BACKGROUND AND OBJECTIVES

Summers and his colleagues note that, because Alzheimer's disease results in part from a dysfunction of acetylcholine neurotransmission, tetrahydroaminoacridine (THA), a centrally acting anticholinesterase inhibitor, may be an effective treatment for Alzheimer's disease. Following this explanation, the authors state, "we report our experience with long-term administration of oral THA to patients in the middle and late stages of suspected Alzheimer's Disease."

Questions

What are the objectives, specific aims, and hypotheses of the study? What previous literature supports these objectives? (Answers are found at the end of the book.)

METHODS

In design, the Summers et al. study is a double-blind crossover clinical trial which began in phase I with 23 subjects 55+ years of age with suspected Alzheimer's disease. The study design and progress of subjects through the study are diagramed in Figure 2–2. The reader is not informed about the source of the subjects.

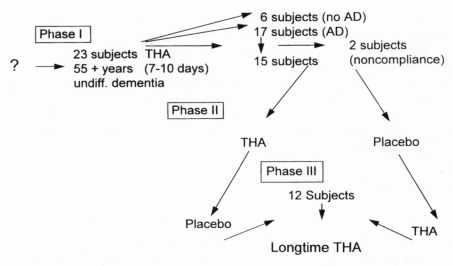

FIGURE 2–2. Study design of the Summers' study (variables). (From Summers et al., 1986.)

All 23 subjects were inpatients, and all were given THA for 7 to 10 days during phase I of the study in order to determine the optimal dose. During phase I, five subjects were diagnosed with conditions other than Alzheimer's disease. Fifteen subjects entered phase II, the placebo-control crossover study. Subjects were randomly assigned to the opposite treatment midway through the trial. Trial subjects then entered phase III, a longer-term time (unspecified) trial on THA.

At baseline of phase II and at 3- and 6-week follow-up the authors measured cognitive impairment, global assessment of function, orientation, names learning, and specific deficits related to Alzheimer's disease using a variety of scales. They divided subjects into moderate and severe Alzheimer's disease based upon assessment at the beginning of phase II.

What concerns do you have about the methods, given this brief description?

RESULTS

The authors found that THA was superior to placebo (statistically significant) on all four measures: Alzheimer's deficit scale, orientation test, the Names Learning Test, and global assessment. The Wilcoxon matched-pair, signed-rank, nonparametric statistical test was used to perform a two-tail test of the null hypothesis that the median test scores in each sample were equal. The differences in baseline vs. treatment (placebo or THA) results for the orientation test are presented for both moderate and severe Alzheimer's disease in Figure 2–3.

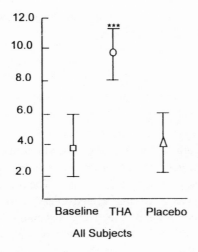

Median values and the 25th to 75th percentile limits are shown for three subgroups
(* denotes P < 0.05, **P < 0.01, and ***P < 0.001).

FIGURE 2–3. Orientation test results. (From Summers et al., 1986.)

THA was superior to placebo in moderate but not severe Alzheimer's disease,
but the authors note that this may be a problem with power (a lack in sufficient
number number of severe cases). THA was also found to be superior to pretreatment on all scales for moderate and on three scales for severe Alzheimer's disease.
No difference was found between pretreatment scores and placebo on any of the
measures.

How would you evaluate these results?

CONCLUSIONS

The authors conclude that in this large study, 10 of 17 subjects demonstrated dramatic objective improvement on psychometric testing. They suggested that improvement might have been due to better assessment of Alzheimer's disease as
well as the use of a THA assay of serum THA levels which permitted higher doses of the drug. For example, subjects without Alzheimer's disease (and who would
not have been expected to respond to THA) were ruled out because of effective
methods of identifying cases prior to the study. They caution, however, that THA
is no more a cure for Alzheimer's disease than levodopa is a cure for Parkinson's
disease. They do suggest, however, that based on these results, THA is a potentially palliative treatment for Alzheimer's disease.

Given what has been presented, how would you evaluate these conclusions based upon the methods and results of the study?

Answers

INTRODUCTION

Other than demonstrating the effectiveness of THA in the treatment of Alzheimer's disease, it is not clear what the authors wish to demonstrate. For example, they do not inform the reader what they mean by effectiveness. The reader later learns in the methods section that they are measuring "effectiveness" using a series of cognitive functioning tests; this definition of effectiveness should be stated clearly in the introduction to the study. The authors do not state any explicit research questions or hypotheses (though later in the study they note, in the methods section, that a statistical test was used to "perform a two-tail test of the null hypothesis that the median test scores in each sample were equal"). The authors' implicit hypothesis is that THA is an effective treatment of Alzheimer's disease when compared to a placebo.

The background for this study is a literature supporting the cholinergic hypothesis for the cognitive dysfunction associated with Alzheimer's disease. A deficit in acetylcholine has been suggested to be associated with decreased cognitive functioning in Alzheimer's patients (though few propose that the actual pathophysiology of Alzheimer's disease is simply a deficit of this neurotransmitter). Therefore the origin of the implicit hypothesis in this study, that THA (an anticholinesterase inhibitor) is an effective treatment for Alzheimer's disease, is clear. Given the literature review, the hypothesis appears reasonable. There is probably enough evidence for a clinical trial if THA is a safe drug—if the drug is not known to be associated with adverse side effects when presented to humans. Alzheimer's disease leads to catastrophic morbidity and there is no known effective therapy. If a drug can potentially delay cognitive decline or improve cognitive functioning in an Alzheimer's patient safely, then such a drug would be welcomed.

METHODS

Many questions about the methods of the study are not answered in the description of the methods provided in the paper. First, other than learning that these subjects were selected from a hospital, it is unclear how they were selected. For example, were these subjects selected randomly or did the investigators simply ask all or a select group of subjects to volunteer for the study? What is the gender and racial/ethnic distribution of these subjects?

Perhaps the most problematic aspect of this study, however, is the lack of clear criteria for who was included in and excluded from the study. Despite noting that they used "standard procedures" for diagnosing subjects and that care in the diagnostic assessment was a key to the success of the clinical trial, the reader is not provided with the criteria used for diagnosing Alzheimer's disease even though considerable testing was performed using laboratory and psychological tests.

Because only 15 subjects completed the study, dividing subjects into two groups (moderate dementia and severe dementia) and comparing them across four measures (global assessment, the orientation test, Names Learning Test, and Alzheimer's deficit scale) provides eight different measures for these 16 subjects. It was likely that some statistically significant result would emerge by chance (see Chapter 12). The consistent and significantly positive results across all tests was dramatic enough, however, to override this methodological problem.

The authors used an appropriate statistical test to compare means: The Wilcoxon Signed-Rank Test determines the difference between two groups in paired samples (and in this study each subject was paired against herself or himself in the crossover design). The test determines the difference for each pair (see Chapter 12).

RESULTS

The report of the results appears appropriate for this study. The authors present the actual data in graphic format. The magnitude of the differences between the treatment and control groups appears meaningful as well as statistically significant. The tables and figures are used effectively in presenting the data, and there appears to be no bias in the figures themselves.

CONCLUSIONS

Despite the statement by the authors that this was a large study of long-term palliative pharmacotherapy with THA, this was a small clinical trial. It is also not clear that the results were "dramatic." As noted above, though the authors conclude that their assessment procedures contributed to better results, it is unclear from the methods and results presented that this in fact was the case. Specifically, without clear diagnostic criteria, it is difficult to determine whether an individual is a "case" of Alzheimer's disease or not, despite the extent of the workup prior to the study (see Chapter 10). If the authors had been more restrained in the conclusions drawn from the results, and more reflective about the methodological flaws, yet had emphasized the interesting findings, most readers with experience in patient-oriented research would have been less critical.

This study is full of methodological flaws and the conclusions are not justified by the methods. Many investigators later commented upon the poor quality of the study. The editors at the *New England Journal of Medicine*, in fact, were probably in a quandary over whether to publish this study. The importance of the disease and the clinically meaningful results, despite the poor methods, encouraged the editors to publish the study. In addition, they believed the study would elicit a significant response from the scientific community, which it did. Large clinical trials, well controlled and well designed, were instituted to study THA in Alzheimer's patients. These trials were forced to be halted for a while because of liver toxicity from THA. The dose of THA was adjusted down. A more careful and larger initial clinical trial by these authors perhaps would have identified the potential for liver toxicity. Lower doses in the larger trial were deemed safe. The result of these clinical trials was the marketing of THA as Cognex in 1994, only 8 years following the publication of the Summers et al. study. The degree of improvement of Alzheimer's disease patients taking THA in these trials was not nearly as great as was initially reported in the Summers study.

NOTES

1. If you have an opportunity, find this article in the library and read it for the exercise above. If not, we have summarized key points in the article about which we pose questions for you similar to the questions we have listed above for studying a study.

2. Unlike other problem sets in this book, the description of the Summers et al. (1986) article is spread across the domains emphasized in the chapter followed by questions relevant to these domains rather than contained entirely at the beginning of the problem set.

REFERENCES

Gunderson J.G., Kolb J.E., Austin V. 1981. The diagnostic interview for borderline patients. *American Journal of Psychiatry* 138: 896–903.

Soloff P.H., Cornelius J., George A., Nathan S., Perel J.M., Ulrich R.F. 1993. Efficacy of phenelzine and haloperidol in borderline personality disorder. *Archives of General Psychiatry* 50: 377–385.

Summers W.K., Majovski L.V., Marsh G.M., Tachiki K., Kling A. 1986. Oral tetrahydroaminoacridine in long-term treatment of senile dementia, Alzheimer type. *New England Journal of Medicine* 315: 1241–1245.

II

STUDY DESIGN

3

LEARNING THE LANGUAGE
OF CLINICAL RESEARCH

OBJECTIVES

- To define common concepts and measures used in clinical research studies.
- To evaluate the appropriateness of measures used to describe the frequency of psychiatric disorders and the associations between risk factors and psychiatric disorders.

CASE EXAMPLE

As part of the Ontario Child Health Study, investigators surveyed early adolescents (n = 726) to assess three types of psychiatric disorders (conduct, attention deficit, and emotional disorders) as they affected substance use in late adolescence. Adolescents (12–16 years of age) and their parents were sampled from households in Ontario, Canada, and they completed structured, self-administered questionnaires. Among the substances assessed were tobacco, alcohol, marijuana, and hard drugs. Both early substance use and conduct disorder were predictors of specific patterns of later substance use. If all conduct disorders could be prevented in this age group and area, the proportions of new marijuana and hard drug use that could be eliminated over 4 years were estimated to be 5.7% and 11.1%, respectively (Boyle et al., 1992).

INTRODUCTION

In order to describe the methods and measures of clinical research studies, investigators use a formal language that unfortunately is often used imprecisely by both the general public and health professionals. Each chapter in this book includes definitions of terms used when conducting or describing specific research methods. This chapter in particular defines and demonstrates the appropriate use of some of the common terms encountered in discussions of epidemiologic research methods. We begin by defining epidemiology broadly as the study of the frequency, distribution, and determinants of health-related states or events in the community at large and in clinical populations or other groups.

A *population* or *target population* is the entire collection of eligible units from which a subset will be drawn for study and to which an investigator would like to generalize the study findings. In most epidemiologic research, the units are individuals or *subjects*, but an investigator might also sample households, hospital records, or institutions. By *population*, epidemiologists do not necessarily mean individuals from a geographically distinct region, but rather a group distinguished by their experience of (i.e., *exposure* to) any characteristic or agent. Thus, one could examine the population of schizophrenic women or the population of families below the poverty line. In the Ontario Child Health Study, of which the example above is a substudy, the population targeted for study included 1,687,200 children aged 4 to 16 years on January 1, 1983, whose usual residence was a household dwelling in Ontario. Of these, 55,100 Ontario children (3.3%) were living on Indian reserves, in collective dwellings, or in dwellings constructed after the 1981 census; they were neither eligible nor included in the study. When all individuals in a population will not be included in the study, the list of individuals or other units from which the sample will be chosen constitutes the *sampling frame*.

A *sample* is a selected subset of the target or study population. The size or number of units in the sample is presented as *n*. As we will see below, the size of the Ontario sample was $n = 726$ adolescents. Samples may be randomly or nonrandomly selected. Random sampling, such as drawing names out of a hat, assumes every person in the population has an equal chance of being selected. Nonrandom sampling occurs when some factor besides chance affects the selection of participants. Nonrandom sampling is sometimes called *purposive* or *purposeful* sampling. Purposeful sampling includes *stratified sampling*. In stratified sampling, the study population is first divided into subgroups by some characteristic or characteristics, such as race or age group, and then a strictly random sample of each subgroup is selected. *Convenience sampling*, in which an easily accessible group of subjects not necessarily representative of the population is studied, is another example of purposeful sampling.

Samples may be drawn from single institutions, multiple institutions, or clinical or population registries. We discuss sampling in greater detail in Chapter 6.

In order to select a representative sample of Ontario households, the investigators in the case example first stratified Ministry of Community and Social Service (MCSS) regions by geographical census areas (based on three categories of population density: large urban, small urban, and rural). As shown in Figure 3–1, households in large urban areas were randomly sampled, whereas households in small urban and rural areas were first grouped into sample areas before being randomly sampled. This was done for the practical reason of reducing high transportation costs associated with surveying less-populated areas.

When the design of a study includes systematic stratified sampling procedures, the analysis of the data may require the use of *poststratification weights* which assign a numerical weight to each participant depending on his or her likelihood of having been selected for the study based on stratification factors such as geography or household size. Sample weights can also adjust the weight of each participant's data to reflect the appropriate demographic characteristics of the target pop-

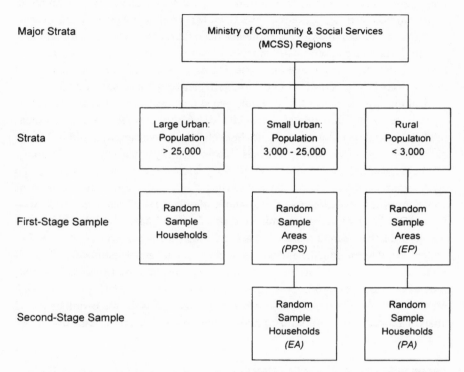

FIGURE 3–1. Design of Ontario Health Study (adapted from Boyle et al., 1987). *PPS* = probability of selection proportional to size; *EP* = equal probability of selection; *EA* = equal allocation; *PA* = proportional allocation.

ulation, e.g., the age and sex distribution of adolescents in the total Ontario population. Use of weights in data analysis is discussed in Chapter 6.

The *effective sample* is comprised of those individuals who have provided complete data for statistical analysis. The effective sample is usually smaller than the
study sample due to incomplete subject responses or attrition over time. In the Ontario study, among children in the age stratum of 12–16 years, 1,302 eligible early adolescents participated in the original Ontario Child Health Study in 1983; of
these 8% (*n* = 100) did not provide complete responses. Of the remaining 1,202,
39.6% did not participate in the follow-up assessment 4 years later. The effective
sample of 726 early adolescents answered questionnaire items about substance use
in 1983 and 1987, and they and their parents completed a problem checklist to assess for conduct disorder and attention deficit disorder in 1983. Data for this subgroup of 726 subjects only were used in the published findings.

An *estimate* is a measurement or a statement about the value of a quantity which
is suspected to incorporate some degree of error. Estimates are inferences about
what is going on in an entire population, based on findings from a sample of that
population. In an attempt to determine the frequency of a disorder in a population,
an investigator can rarely examine every single person in that population, so he or
she samples the population and estimates the extent of a disorder or its relationship to a risk factor based on that sample. Moreover, even in the most representative subsample of the population, some degree of bias is at work—e.g., affected
persons may be erroneously counted as unaffected (or vice versa), or there may be
clinical disagreement about who should and should not be counted as affected.

In this example, the authors estimated the extent of substance abuse and mental disorders among Ontario early adolescents based on a subgroup of all Ontario
early adolescents who were both accessible and willing to participate in the study.
Of the approximately 650,000 Ontario early adolescents in the population, 726
adolescents were selected for the study. Thus, the investigators drew conclusions
about an entire population based on a sample of only 0.1% of that population. Adolescents in the study were determined to be using marijuana if either their checklist score or their parent's checklist score for marijuana use was positive. Other
methods of determining marijuana use might well change the estimate. The validity of an estimated measure depends on the implementation of rigorous methodological and analytic procedures. In later chapters, common sources of estimation
error and bias in cohort and case-control studies as well as the methodological and
analytic procedures for minimizing and quantifying their magnitude are discussed.

PROPORTIONS, RATES, AND RISK

Definitions of the most commonly estimated measures are listed in Table 3–1. A
common estimate of the frequency of occurrence of a disorder in a population is

TABLE 3–1. Common measures used in clinical research studies

Proportions, rates, and risk
- Point prevalence: the number of cases of a disorder in a population at a specified point in time
- Period prevalence: the number of cases of a disorder in a population during a specified period of time
- Cumulative incidence: the probability that an individual will experience an event during a specified period of time
- Incidence rate: the proportion of all unaffected persons at risk of a disorder who become affected in a specified population during a specified period of time
- Mortality rate: the proportion of a population that dies during a specified period of time
- Case fatality rate: the proportion of persons affected by a disorder who die during a specified period of time
- Crude rate: the proportion of an entire population affected during a specified period of time
- Category-specific rate: the proportion of a subgroup of the population, e.g., gender, race, or age subgroups, affected during a specified period of time
- Adjusted rate: the average proportion of persons affected in the population over a specified period of time, weighted according to category-specific rates
- Risk: the probability that an individual at risk of a disorder will become affected during a specified period of time

Differences and ratios
- Rate difference for the exposed: the absolute difference in the rates of affected persons in an exposed and an unexposed population
- Rate ratio: the ratio of incidence rates of a disorder for two groups in a population who differ in their exposure to a risk factor
- Risk ratio: the ratio of probabilities of developing a disorder for two groups in a population who differ in their exposure to a risk factor
- Attributable risk percent for the population: the proportion of the occurrence of a disorder that could be eliminated if the exposure to the risk factor were prevented

prevalence. Although sometimes called a prevalence rate, *prevalence* is a simple proportion, and is calculated as follows:

$$\text{Prevalence} = \frac{\text{number of individuals affected by a given disorder}}{\text{number of individuals in the population}}$$

Affected individuals may be counted at a designated point in time (point prevalence) or during a relatively brief period of time (period prevalence). Therefore, prevalence measures the probability that an individual in the population will have a disorder at that time. For example, among 726 early adolescents in Ontario in 1983, 53 reported regular alcohol or tobacco use, 18 the regular use of alcohol or tobacco and marijuana, and 17 the regular use of alcohol or tobacco, marijuana, and hard drugs during the past 12 months. Therefore, the estimated 1-year period prevalence of these patterns of substance abuse was .073, .025, and .023, respectively. Lifetime prevalence is the probability that an individual in the population at a given time has ever been affected by the disorder; it is a useful measure for remittent disorders such as major depression.

Incidence density, unlike prevalence, is a true rate that measures change per unit time. The incidence density (*ID*), also called the incidence rate or hazard rate, is one of two measures of incidence used in epidemiologic research. The incidence density is the average rate at which persons fall ill (numerator) during a given follow-up period of specified duration in a population at risk of falling ill (denominator):

$$ID = I / PT$$

where I = number of new cases and PT is person-time (expressed as person-months, person-years, etc.).

For example, among the 582 early adolescents who were not substance users in 1983, 174 were using tobacco or alcohol, 67 were using tobacco or alcohol plus marijuana, and 25 were using tobacco or alcohol plus marijuana plus hard drugs in 1987. The average annual incidence rate of tobacco or alcohol use among Ontario adolescents was 174 / (582 × 4) or approximately .075 new users/year. The estimated four-year *incidence density* or *incidence rate* or *hazard rate* for each of the three respective patterns of substance use, i.e., the proportion of all participants who were not users in 1983 who began substance use between 1983 and 1987, was .299, .115, and .043.

Cumulative incidence (CI), on the other hand, is an estimate of *risk* or probability that an individual will become a new case during the follow-up period, such as the probability that an individual will experience a major depressive episode in one's lifetime or experience a relapse in major depression within 12 months following a remission. Cumulative incidence is not a rate in that it does not measure change over time, although cumulative incidence has the following relationship to the incidence rate:

$$CI = 1 - e^{[-(\text{mean per-person incidence rate} \times \text{length of observation})]}$$

where e is the base of the natural logarithm (2.71828), where the incidence rate is calculated for the individual rather than for a population group, and where the incidence rate and the observation period are measured in equivalent units of time.

Measures of incidence, whether rates or risk, are only as accurate as the *surveillance* of the subjects has been over the course of the study. Follow-up of every individual for a period of years is rarely possible, due to deaths from competing causes, dropouts, and other losses to follow-up. Person-time of follow-up is most accurately calculated from the sum of the days (or months or years) that each person in the study was monitored prior to being censored. *Censoring* a subject involves truncating the time contributed by a given subject to that subject's total observation period because (1) the event of interest has occurred; (2) the subject was lost to follow-up because of refusal to continue, a residential move beyond the surveillance area, death due to other causes, etc.; or (3) the study ended.

To illustrate the differences among these measures of the occurrence of disorders, hypothetical data from a longitudinal study of the course of depression are presented in Figure 3–2. Forty-five patients with major depression (MD) experienced a remission of their symptoms within 6 months of an index episode and were scheduled to be interviewed every 6 months following remission to 48 months beyond the index episode. All 45 patients were administered the Center for Epidemiologic Studies-Depression (CES-D) scale (Radloff, 1977) at the 6- and 12-month interviews. Subsequently, individual patients left the study over time until only five subjects remained in the study 48 months after the index episode.

Using these data, investigators might wish to estimate the probability of reporting significant depressive symptomatology at any time during the first year following remission (1-year period prevalence). Of 45 patients, 12 reported high CES-D scores at either the 6-month or 12-month interview, for a 1-year period prevalence of depression of .267 among patients with a previously remitted episode. Thus, the probability of experiencing significant depressive symptoms within 12 months of a remission was 26.7% in this population.

These data could also be used to estimate the incidence density of relapse in the 3 years following remission of MD. Of the 45 patients in remission, 29 experienced a relapse of significant symptoms at some time during the 3 years such that an average incidence rate of relapse might be calculated as 29 / (45 × 3) or 21.5 relapses/year/100 persons. However, because not all 45 patients contributed 3 years of observation, a more precise estimate of the incidence density would take into account the varying lengths of follow-up time under observation prior to a relapse or loss to follow-up. From Figure 3–2, one observes an accumulated total of 900 months of follow-up before all patients had been censored, for an incidence rate of (29 relapses / 900 person-months) × (12 months) × (100 persons) or 38.7 relapses/year/100 patients. The probability that a patient with remitted MD would relapse within 1 year would be:

$$1 - e^{[-(.032 \text{ relapses per person per month} \times 12 \text{ months})]} \text{ or } .321 \text{ or } 32.1\%$$

When there is little attrition over time from the sample of individuals being observed for new events (as occurs when observation periods are short), or when incidence rates are very low (as occurs with rare disorders), the observed incidence density in the patient population will closely approximate the cumulative incidence (or estimated risk to an individual patient). This is rarely the case because losses to follow-up accumulate in most psychiatric studies due to deaths, refusals to participate, migration beyond the surveillance area, and other factors. These losses remove potential new cases from the population at risk and distort the mea-

Time Elapsed (Months from Remission)

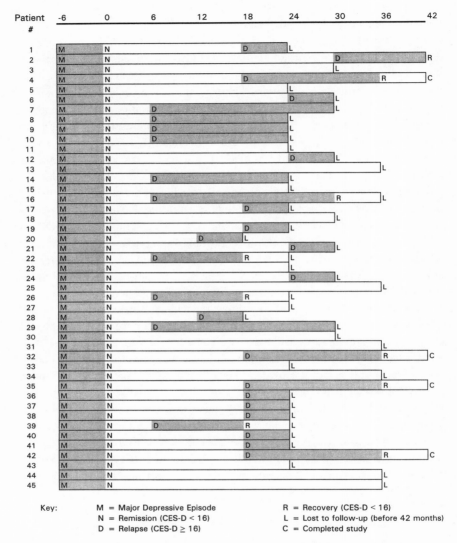

FIGURE 3–2. Relapse and recovery following remission of an index major depressive episode (MDE), in months.

sure of event occurrence. In the example of relapse of MD, simply multiplying the average per-person monthly incidence density of .032 by 12 months of observation would yield a spuriously higher probability of relapse (.387) than the actual probability (.321). The various methods for calculating risk and the study design assumptions on which they are based are described more completely in Kleinbaum et al. (1982).

Other types of rates are mortality (death) rates and case fatality rates. A *mortality rate* is the proportion of a population that dies during a specified period. For example, in 1987 there were a total of 8,139 alcohol-related motor vehicle crash deaths among an estimated population of 38,252,000 persons aged 15–24 (U.S. National Highway Traffic Safety Administration, 1988), for an average mortality rate of 21.3 deaths per 100,000 at-risk persons per year. (Also, see Chapter 7 for use of mortality rates in the Stirling County Study.)

A *case fatality rate* is the proportion of persons affected by a disorder who die within a specified time. For example, if there were 18.5 million persons in the U.S. who abused alcohol and 105,000 died of alcohol-related causes in a given year, the case fatality rate for alcohol abuse would be six deaths per 1,000 affected persons per year.

Rates may be presented as crude, category-specific, or adjusted rates. *Crude rates* are based on changes over time in an entire population; *category-specific rates* are based on changes over time in subgroups of the population—such as gender, race, or age subgroups. *Adjusted rates* are weighted averages of category-specific rates. Each kind of rate is useful for specific purposes. For example, the U.S. Public Health Service disease prevention and health promotion effort *Healthy People 2000* has targeted the age-adjusted U.S. homicide rate of 8.5 per 100,000 (for year 1987) for reduction to 7.2 per 100,000 by the year 2000 (U.S. National Center for Health Statistics, 1991). The 1987 age-adjusted rate is a weighted average of that year's homicide rates for all age categories. Age-specific annual homicide rates for the same year varied widely, with low rates among children under 5 and the elderly (3.4 and 4.6 per 100,000, respectively) and much higher rates (15.3 per 100,000) among young adults (U.S. National Center for Health Statistics, 1990, 1993; U.S. Bureau of the Census, 1993). The program has targeted for intervention specific age, race, and gender subgroups where prevention might significantly reduce the rate of homicide between years 1987 and 2000, e.g., among spouses aged 15–34 (from 1.7 to 1.4 homicides per 100,000/year); among black women aged 15–34 (from 20.0 to 16.0 homicides per 100,000/year); and among black men aged 15–34 (from 90.5 to 72.4 homicides per 100,000/year). The age-adjusted national homicide rate provides a useful estimate permitting comparisons of the U.S. population to those other nations, while the age-specific rates can be used to target public health programs to reduce excess risk in specific population subgroups.Although the above example deals with mortality rates, other rates, such as those measuring incidence of psychiatric disorders, can also be expressed as crude, category-specific, or adjusted rates.

DIFFERENCES AND RATIOS

The primary task of epidemiology is to compare rates or risks of a disorder between two groups in a population that differ in their exposure to a characteristic or agent. An exposure thought to raise the risk of the disorder is a *risk factor*; one thought to lower the risk of the disorder is a *protective factor*. One needs efficient and informative summary measures to make such comparisons between or across groups. The measures most often employed are the rate difference, the rate ratio, and the risk ratio.

The *rate difference* expresses the magnitude of the difference in frequency of a disorder between two groups during a time period. Because the comparison is usually between exposed and unexposed groups, the rate difference is specified *for the exposed* to avoid confusion with the population estimates described below.

The rate difference for the exposed is calculated from incidence density. In the Ontario example (Boyle et al., 1992), the 4-year incidence of new marijuana use among previous nonusers was 38.7 per 100 early adolescents with a conduct disorder (exposed) and 17.6 per 100 without a conduct disorder (unexposed). The rate difference for the use of marijuana among adolescents with a positive vs. a negative history of conduct disorder is (38.7–17.6) or 21.1 per 100 early adolescents at risk per 4 years.

The *incidence density ratio* or *rate ratio* is another common measure of association used to compare the rates of a disorder across groups who were and were not exposed to a factor of interest. The Ontario investigators calculated the incidence density ratio for beginning marijuana use among early adolescent nonusers between 12 and 16 years of age by dividing the incidence rate for the exposed group (38.7) by that for the unexposed group (17.6). They found that early adolescents with positive history of conduct disorder had (38.7 / 17.6) or approximately 2.2 times the rate of beginning marijuana use compared to those with a negative history.

A *risk ratio* compares the relative risk of two cumulative incidences or probabilities, e.g., the risk that an early adolescent with conduct disorder will initiate the use of marijuana compared to the risk that an early adolescent with no conduct disorder will initiate the use of marijuana. An example of calculating relative risk is included in Chapter 7. An *odds ratio* compares the likelihood of having been exposed to a risk factor among persons who have a disorder to the likelihood of exposure among persons who do not have the disorder.

The proportion of exposed cases that are due to the risk factor can be estimated from the incidence density ratio (*IDR*). This *etiologic fraction for the exposed* is calculated as:

$$(IDR - 1) / IDR, \text{ or } (2.2 - 1) / 2.2 = .545$$

Thus, more than half of new use of marijuana in the study was associated with a positive history of conduct disorder.

Attributable risk percent for the population is a useful tool for estimating the proportion of the occurrence of a disorder that could be eliminated if the exposure to the risk factor were prevented. The measure of association between a risk factor and a disorder in two exposure groups depends on the ratio of rates between the two groups as well as the prevalence of the risk factor in the population. The attributable risk percent for the population is calculated as:

$$\frac{(\text{Prevalence of the exposure}) \times (\text{rate ratio} - 1)}{1 + [(\text{Prevalence of the exposure}) \times (\text{rate ratio} - 1)]}$$

In the Ontario example, the prevalence of conduct disorder among early adolescents was just over 5.5% (40 / 726). Thus, the percentage of onset of marijuana use over 4 years by early adolescents in Ontario which might be eliminated if all conduct disorders in this age group could be prevented would be:

$$\frac{(0.055) \times (2.20 - 1)}{1 + [(0.055) \times (2.20 - 1)]} = 6.2\%$$

The attributable risk percent for the population is a particularly relevant measure for calculating the potential value of programs which target the reduction of risk factors associated with chronic mental disorders, especially when those disorders are relatively rare and also may have multiple causes. Where a risk factor for a disorder is relatively rare, it cannot account for a large proportion of that disorder unless it is very nearly a necessary condition for that disorder.

Two measures are discussed in more detail elsewhere in this text. Relative risk is discussed in Chapter 7 and the *exposure odds ratio* in Chapter 8.

Problem Set

Bruce et al. (1994) examined the effects of nine *DSM-III* Axis I psychiatric disorders on the risk of mortality over a 9-year period among New Haven County, CT, middle-aged and elderly adults. This study, as part of the Epidemiologic Catchment Area Program (ECA), used the Diagnostic Interview Schedule (DIS) (Robins et al., 1981) to identify cases of each disorder. In 1980, a sample of adults 18 years and old-

TABLE 3–2. Baseline psychiatric diagnosis and 9-year mortality risk for New Haven ECA Study respondents aged 40 and older: relative risk estimated by proportional hazards model and adjusted for sex and age

| | | DECEASED | | ADJUSTED RELATIVE | CHI-SQUARE ANALYSIS | |
DIS DIAGNOSIS	TOTAL	N	%	RISK	χ^2 (df = 1)	p
Total	3,560	1,194	33.5			
Major depression						
Recent	67	26	38.8	2.01	12.36	.0004
Past	50	13	26.0	1.54	2.40	.12
Alcohol abuse / dependence						
Recent	64	20	31.3	1.79	6.50	.01
Past	131	50	38.1	1.47	21.05	.0001

Data from Bruce et al., (1994), Table 2.

er was drawn from a total adult population served by the Connecticut Mental Health Center, which included primarily residents of the New Haven–West Haven Standard Metropolitan Area (SMA) (Leaf et al., 1991). The sampling procedures included stratification by households (from public utility listings) and by psychiatric, nursing home, and correctional institutions (from city directories) (Holzer et al., 1985; Leaf et al., 1985; see Chapter 6 for additional information on ECA sampling methods). Of the approximately 300,000 eligible respondents, 6,538 were invited to participate, and 5,034 (77%) consented to an interview. Few adults younger than 40 died during the 9 years of follow-up, so only those subjects who were 40 years of age and older were included in this study, resulting in an effective sample of 3,560 (Bruce et al., 1994).

Of the 3,560 subjects, 526 men and 668 women were confirmed to be deceased over the 9 years of follow-up; 889 men and 1,455 women were confirmed to be alive in 1989 and information was unavailable for the remaining 22 subjects. Table 3–2 presents the frequencies and percentages of recent (one-year) and lifetime frequencies of (DIS-diagnosed) major depression and alcohol abuse/dependence in the New Haven ECA as well as the estimated risk of mortality to affected individuals compared to those not affected.

Questions

1. What are the average annual mortality rates, separately, for men and women aged 40 and older in the New Haven–West Haven SMA?

2. Would you expect that mortality rates derived from this sample would be higher, lower, or similar if they were age-adjusted to include adults 18–39 years of age?

3. What is the risk of dying over a 9-year period, separately, for the average man and woman aged 40 and over in the New Haven–West Haven SMA?

4. Calculate the average annual mortality rate difference between men and women.

5. Calculate the average annual mortality rate ratio of men to women.

6. Calculate the 9-year mortality risk ratio of men to women.

7. Calculate the attributable mortality risk percent to the population of (a) all recent episodes of major depressive episode (MDE) and (b) lifetime alcohol abuse/dependence.

8. If MDE were more common in this population (e.g., 10% prevalence), how would that affect the attributable mortality risk percent to the population?

Answers

1. Average annual mortality rates:

$$\{\ [\ 526\ /\ (526 + 889)\ ]\ \div 9\ \}\ \times 1{,}000 = 41.3 \text{ deaths }/1{,}000 \text{ men / year}$$

$$\{\ [\ 668\ /\ (668 + 1{,}455)\ ]\ \div 9\ \}\ \times 1{,}000 = 35.0 \text{ deaths }/1{,}000 \text{ women / year}$$

2. The estimated rates would likely be lower, because mortality is less prevalent among adults 18–39.

3. Nine-year mortality risk:

$$1 - e^{[-(41.3\ /\ 1{,}000)\ \times\ 9 \text{ years})]} = .31 \text{ for men}$$

$$1 - e^{[-(35.0\ /\ 1{,}000)\ \times\ 9 \text{ years})]} = .27 \text{ for women}$$

4. Average annual mortality rate difference between men and women aged 40 and over =

$$41.3 - 35.0 = 6.3 \text{ deaths }/1{,}000 \text{ persons / year}$$

5. Average annual mortality rate ratio (men : women) =

$$41.3\ /\ 35.0 = 1.18$$

6. Nine-year-mortality risk ratio (men : women) =

$$.31\ /\ .27 = 1.15$$

These calculations indicate that an average estimated 41.3 of 100,000 New Haven–West Haven male residents and 35.0 of 100,000 of female residents over 40 years of age died during each year of follow-up. The probability of death over 9 years of follow-up in this age range was 31% for men and 27% for women. Each year among each 1,000 men and women, approximately six more men than women died, and the annual mortality rate was 18% higher among men than among women. The "average" man in this population had a 15% higher probability of dying over the 9 years than did the "average" woman.

7. Calculations of attributable mortality risk percent to the population:

(a) for recent MDE:

$$[(67 / 3,560) \times (2.01 - 1.00)] / \{1 + [(67 / 3,560) \times (2.01 - 1.00)] \} = 1.9\%$$

(b) for lifetime alcohol abuse/dependence:

$$[(131 / 3,560) \times (1.47 - 1.00)] / \{1 + [(131 / 3,560) \times (1.47 - 1.00)] \} = 1.7\%$$

Thus, of the deaths from all causes occurring over nine years among New Haven adults aged 40 years and older, 1.9% could be prevented if the onset of all major depressive episodes within a year of baseline measurement could be prevented, and 1.7% could be prevented if lifetime alcohol abuse and dependence could be eliminated.

8. If the prevalence of recent major depressive episodes was 10% instead of just under 2%, this change would considerably increase the attributable mortality risk among the population, as demonstrated by these calculations:

$$[(356 / 3,560) \times (2.01 - 1.00)] / \{1 + [(356 / 3,560) \times (2.01 - 1.00)] \} = 9.2\%$$

REFERENCES

Boyle M.H., Offord D.R., Hofmann H.G., Catlin G.P., Byles J.A., Cadman D.T., Crawford J.W., Links P.S., Rae-Grant N.I., Szatmari P. 1987. Ontario Child Health Study: I. Methodology. *Archives of General Psychiatry* 44: 826–831.

Boyle M.H., Offord D.R., Racine Y.A., Szatmari P., Fleming J.E., Links P.S. 1992. Predicting substance abuse in late adolescence: results from the Ontario Child Health Study Follow-Up. *American Journal of Psychiatry* 149: 761–767.

Bruce M.L., Leaf P.J., Rozal G.P.M., Florio L., Hoff R.A. 1994. Psychiatric status and 9-year mortality data in the New Haven Epidemiologic Catchment Area Study. *American Journal of Psychiatry* 151: 716–721.

Holzer C.E. III, Spitznagel E., Jordan K.B., Timbers D.M., Kessler L.G., Anthony J.C. 1985. Sampling the household population. In *Epidemiologic Field Methods in Psychiatry: The NIMH Epidemiologic Catchment Area Program* (eds. Eaton W.W., Kessler L.G.), pp. 23–48. Orlando, FL: Academic Press.

Kleinbaum D.G., Kupper L.L., Morgenstern H. 1982. *Epidemiologic Research: Principles and Quantitative Methods*. New York: Van Nostrand Reinhold.

Leaf P.J., German P.S., Spitznagel E., George L.K., Landsverk J., Windle C.D. 1985. Sampling: the institutional survey. In *Epidemiologic Field Methods in Psychiatry: The*

NIMH Epidemiologic Catchment Area Program (eds. Eaton W.W., Kessler L.G.), pp. 49–66. Orlando, FL: Academic Press.

Leaf P.J., Myers J.K., McEvoy L.T. 1991. Procedures used in the Epidemiologic Catchment Area Study. In *Psychiatric Disorders in America: The Epidemiologic Catchment Area Study* (eds. Robins L.N., Regier D.A.), pp. 11–32. New York: Free Press.

Radloff L.S. 1977. The CES-D scale: a self-report depression scale for research in the general population. *Applied Psychological Measurement* 1: 385–401.

Robins L.N., Helzer J.E., Croughan J., Ratcliff K.S. 1981. National Institute of Mental Health Diagnostic Interview Schedule: its history, characteristics, and validity. *Archives of General Psychiatry* 38: 381–389.

U.S. Bureau of the Census. 1993. *Current Population Reports* (P25–1095), *U.S. Population Estimates by Age, Sex, Race, and Hispanic Origin: 1980 to 1991*. Washington, DC: U.S. Government Printing Office.

U.S. National Center for Health Statistics. 1990. *Vital Statistics of the United States—1987. Vol. II, Mortality, Part A.* DHHS Pub. No. (PHS) 90–1101. Washington, DC: Public Health Service.

U.S. National Center for Health Statistics. 1991. *Healthy People 2000: National Health Promotion and Disease Prevention Objectives.* DHHS Pub. No. (PHS) 91–50212. Washington, DC: Public Health Service.

U.S. National Center for Health Statistics. 1993. *Health United States, 1992.* Hyattsville, MD: Public Health Service.

U.S. National Highway Traffic Safety Administration. 1988. *Fatal Accident Reporting System, 1987.* DOT-HS-807 360. Washington, DC: U.S. Department of Transportation.

4

SINGLE-SUBJECT DESIGN

OBJECTIVES

- To understand the purpose (and types of) single subject design as an investigative method in clinical psychiatric research.
- To critique both the relevance and content of the types of single-subject design for use by clinicians and clinical investigators.
- To understand and critique case studies/case conferences.
- To understand and critique single-subject time-series design.
- To understand and critique ecologic psychological design.

CASE EXAMPLE 1 (CASE STUDY/CASE CONFERENCE)

Sobel and colleagues (1996) presented the case of a 33-year-old African-American veteran who was admitted to the hospital with a diagnosis of chronic paranoid schizophrenia. (This case presentation was published as one of the series of "clinical case conferences" recently added to each issue of the *American Journal of Psychiatry*.) The authors provided detailed information about the current symptoms and past history of this patient and emphasized that though the patient met diagnostic criteria for paranoid schizophrenia, he did not display the classic Bleulerian symptoms of autism. On the contrary, they noted that the patient was "engaging and relates well to others." The patient was admitted to the hospital following an episode of severe agitation and social withdrawal and experienced command auditory hallucinations from a delusional companion.

The case presentation was followed by a transcribed discussion led by Robert Cancro, an expert in the diagnosis and treatment of schizophrenia. As Dr. Cancro noted, the case highlighted that not everyone who is psychotic is best thought of as experiencing a variant of schizophrenia. He commented that the patient had adequate ability to relate to others and to maintain attachments, and, with treatment, recovered within a short period of time. This patient should be considered representative of an individual with limited resources who, when experiencing excessive anxiety and rage, may regress into a severe psychotic state yet recover quickly. Such patients should not be conceptualized or diagnosed as schizophrenic.

CASE EXAMPLE 2 (SINGLE-SUBJECT TIME-SERIES DESIGN)

Because of an association with subjective emotional and cardiovascular effects, Volkow and colleagues (1996) performed positron emission tomography (PET) to study the pharmacokinetics of methylphenidate in the human brain over time. Intravenous injections of methylphenidate at 0.5 mg/kg were administered to four subjects who were tested. Each subject showed similar uptake of the labeled methylphenidate into the brain and a similar decrease in binding of methylphenidate in the basal ganglia after the dose of methylphenidate (Fig. 4–1). Restlessness and changes in systolic blood pressure and heart rate followed a temporal course which paralleled closely the pharmacokinetics of methylphenidate in the brain. In contrast, however, methylphenidate induced a "high," anxiety, and changes in diastolic blood pressure which decreased rapidly after injection despite long-lasting binding of the drug in the brain. The authors plotted the perception of a "high," anxiety, restlessness, diastolic blood pressure, systolic blood pressure, and heart rate with time across the abscissa as they did uptake and concentration in the brain. Therefore some subjective symptoms, such as restlessness, were temporarily associated with the uptake and concentration of methylphenidate, but other subjective emotions, such as a "high," were not.

CASE STUDIES/CASE CONFERENCES

Single-subject design can be divided into three broad categories based upon the methodology employed and the nature of the subject investigated: case study/case conference, time series design, and ecologic psychological design. The above examples represent the first two of these categories. Single-subject design has a unique role in psychiatric research, both for its relevance to overall case management and for the initial exploration of phenomena such as pharmacokinetic responses to a medication. In recent years, however, psychiatrists and clinical investigators have tended to distrust these methods. A review of a recent issue of the

% Dose/CC Tissue

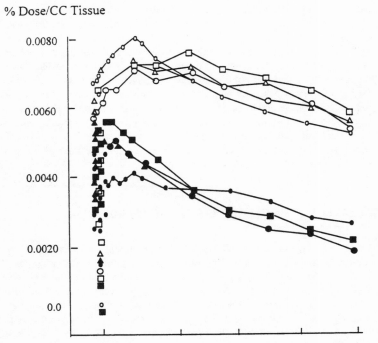

FIGURE 4–1. Individual time activity curves for rate of uptake of [^{11}C]methylphenidate in basal ganglia (open symbols) and cerebellum (closed symbols), expressed as percent injected dose per cubic centimeter of tissue. Each symbol denotes a different subject with the corresponding paired parameter (denoted as open or closed). The time–activity curves for the absolute uptake of [^{11}C]methylphenidate as well as for the change in the basal ganglia to cerebellar ratios after administration did not differ between the subjects. (From Volkow et al., 1996.)

American Journal of Psychiatry will reveal case studies among the "Letters to the Editor." The *Journal* has adopted the policy that the appropriate place for case reports is in a Letter to the Editor, for a single-case study is not quantitative clinical research. Typically, a case of particular interest is described in some detail and followed by a brief commentary. A common rationale for presenting a case is to report a unique therapeutic or side effect of a medication, previously unreported, thus informing clinicians to be vigilant about this potential response and perhaps guiding clinical investigators to pursue new clinical trials or monitor medications based on such case reports. For example, a series of isolated case reports about the potential of fluoxetine to cause suicidal ideation (and perhaps precipitate a suicide attempt) led to extensive epidemiologic surveillance of persons prescribed fluox-etine some years ago.

A clinical case conference, such as example 1, is typically prepared for teach-ing purposes. It differs from a case study in that the primary goal is education about more common problems and their management rather than reporting unique clin-ical findings. Its educational value often derives from the interaction between the author's objective presentation of the "data" about the individual under consider-ation and the expert consultants' reflection upon these data. For example, the So-bel and colleagues study was reported and discussed to educate psychiatrists about the conceptualization and diagnosis of schizophrenia within the context of our cur-rent diagnostic nomenclature.

How can case studies be of value as an educational technique? Neale and Lieber (1973) suggest four possible ways:

- A prototypical example to illustrate some behavior of a patient or response of a patient to a particular environmental stimulus.
- A demonstration of a particular diagnostic or therapeutic procedure.
- A detailed account of a rare or unusual phenomenon.
- A means to challenge an alleged universal aspect of a particular theoretical position.

Case example 1 illustrates the fourth possibility. In this case presentation, an in-dividual who had been labeled as a chronic paranoid schizophrenic was evaluated in detail by a world expert in the field of schizophrenia. Doctor Cancro empha-sized in this case conference that the patient exhibited symptoms that Kurt Schrei-der described as being typically associated with schizophrenia: audible thoughts, voices, and delusional perceptions (Schneider, 1959). However, he went on to note that

> there is an underlying characteristic which has permeated virtually all concepts of schizophrenia, namely a blunting of affect and autism. This patient did not fill either of these criteria and therefore, though he "in practice" fills the criteria for para-noid schizophrenia according the *DSM-IV*, he "in theory" should not be considered schizophrenic.

Prototypical examples of cases are rarely found in peer-reviewed journals (ex-cept as educational case reports) but are frequently placed in textbooks to illustrate the typical clinical picture of a particular psychiatric disorder, such as major de-pression or panic disorder. Yet peer-reviewed journals are replete with case stud-ies illustrating new methods and procedures. Most of the methods reported today involve new uses of medications to treat certain symptoms. They are not, howev-er, evidence whose existence allows clinicians to adopt the uses reported in routine practice. Therefore editors of journals are at times unlikely to publish case studies for fear a case study will be accepted as sufficient evidence to institute a new treatment.

Another frequent use of case reports is to provide detailed accounts of rare or unusual phenomena. In fact, one of the authors of this book in his first publication described a paranoid psychotic reaction in an individual who was taking phentazocine, a frequently prescribed narcotic analgesic at the time (Blazer and Haller, 1975). These types of case reports generally are used to document potential side effects of medications. To our knowledge, this case report of phentazocine psychosis (the first such report to be published) led to the statement, "patients receiving therapeutic doses of phentazocine have experienced hallucinations (usually visual), disorientation and confusion which have cleared spontaneously within a period of hours," in the *Physicians' Desk Reference* (1994).

What are the potential problems associated with case studies? First, and foremost, clinicians and clinical investigators must not overgeneralize from case studies. The virtual disappearance of case studies as regular articles in peer-reviewed journals reflects a concern about overgeneralization and potential bias resulting from such generalization. The comparison of a group of cases and controls is a far better means to demonstrate the existence of phenomena or to provide evidence that a particular therapeutic intervention is effective. Clinical trials provide the strongest basis for major clinical decisions. Case studies should instead be considered the stimulus for further research or vigilance about the phenomena reported. Nevertheless, clinicians gain considerable experience with their own patients and develop intuitive approaches to therapy based upon these cases. Case studies supplement these individual experiences and are therefore attractive to the practicing clinician.

The most valuable case reports and conferences "make a point," usually a single point. The focus of both the presentation and discussion should emphasize that point. It is imperative for the author of a case history to make explicit, within the first few sentences, why it is being reported. For example, in Sobel et al. (1996), the focus is on the notion that some persons labeled as schizophrenic can be diagnosed incorrectly because of the prominence of some symptoms of schizophrenia. If a case is reported because "this is an interesting case," the report is frequently flawed because it is too diffuse. The "interest" of the clinician therefore flaws the case report because the clinician does not specify what is interesting.

A detailed description of the nuances of a therapeutic procedure may require a detailed description of the patient. For example, the psychoanalytic literature is replete with detailed case histories used to illustrate both theory and technique, such as Freud's in depth description of the case of Anna O (Twemblow and Warnock, 1977). Nevertheless, the use of detailed narratives of a case to provide guidance regarding techniques of a particular therapeutic approach has been received with skepticism by many nonpsychoanalytic psychiatrists. When the techniques of interpersonal psychotherapy, were first reported, for example, the authors focused their report on generic aspects of the therapy rather than detailed case examples (Klerman et al., 1984).

SINGLE-SUBJECT TIME-SERIES DESIGN

A single-subject time-series design is used to identify a "pattern" but assumes that the pattern can be abstracted from data derived from a single subject (or at most a group of subjects too small in number to apply statistical analysis of group trends). The rationale is that human beings have similar responses to certain stimuli, such as being given a medication, and some generalizations can derive from the report of even one subject.

Case example 2 by Volkow and colleagues (1996) illustrates single subject time-series design. The investigators studied four subjects, and their essential findings came from identifying a response to a stimulus, as seen in Figure 4–1. Time-series design is descriptive and illustrative. The Volkow et al. study is characteristic of many time-series designs in that the authors obtained baseline data, introduced a "stimulus" (in this case methylphenidate), and then recorded the response to the stimulus across a number of parameters (heart rate, blood pressure, experience of a "high," and anxiety).

Time-series design is often inherent to usual psychiatric therapy. A depressed patient referred to a psychiatrist, for example, might be evaluated for symptoms with a scale such as the Hamilton Depression Rating Scale and then given an antidepressant, such as fluoxetine, 20 mg p.o. q.d. The psychiatrist would follow that patient to determine if there is a change in symptoms from baseline at intervals after baseline (such as 1 week, 3 weeks, 6 weeks, 3 months, and 6 months). If there is no change, or the psychiatrist believes the change is not clinically significant, he or she might withdraw the medication and use the same scale for 1 or 2 more weeks to determine if there is a worsening of symptoms. In this way, the most effective treatment can be tailored and monitored for an individual patient. The use of rating scales when treating a psychiatric patient is not considered "clinical research," yet it illustrates time-series design as it is most often employed.

In reporting a time-series design, the data are usually presented in a graph with time plotted along the abscissa and the observation (or observations) of interest plotted along the ordinate. In Figure 4–1, for example, the rate of uptake of methylphenidate in the basal ganglia is plotted along the ordinate and time along the abscissa.

Time-series design may be of value when traditional experimental design is not appropriate or feasible. It provides a careful documentation of fluctuations in an outcome variable over time (Gottman and McFall, 1972). For example, the fluctuation of depressive symptoms from one day to the next (not to mention from one part of the day to another) is rarely captured in typical outcome studies or clinical trials (such as the Psychobiology of Depression Study described in Chapter 7). Time-series design can also provide a source of material for testing a hypothesis about an individual patient, whether that material can be generalized or not. Consider, for example, an older woman who is experiencing memory difficulties. Family members note that she becomes excessively agitated during the evenings, and the psychiatrist asks the family to plot the woman's agitation for a number of days in relation to events in the household. Agitation is documented to increase each day as dinner time approaches. The psychiatrist then may assume that the problems of continuing to prepare meals and becoming confused during the process are precipitating the woman's anxiety and agitation. Time-series design may also be useful when a control group is not practical. In other words, a time series permits an individual patient to serve as his or her control (as in taking a drug and then stopping the drug).

ECOLOGIC PSYCHOLOGICAL STUDY

A type of single-case study that differs from case study and time-series designs is the ecologic psychological study. The "single subject" in this design is not a person, but rather a "setting," such as a hospital. Ecologic psychological studies rarely appear in the mainstream psychiatric literature today, yet they had an important role at midcentury. One of the best-known examples (1961) is the account by Irving Goffman of a mental hospital where he was a "participant-observer" for over a year. In his book *Asylums*, Goffman described virtually every aspect of life in this hospital and emphasized what the environment "makes of the inmates."

Robert Barker and his colleagues (1968) took a different approach to ecologic psychological study. They set up carefully detailed studies of natural settings, such as the waiting room of a psychiatric clinic on a Thursday afternoon from 1 o'clock to 5 o'clock. An observer recorded in minute detail every event he observed during this time period. The researchers determined whether certain "action patterns" took place in these settings, such as an aesthetic action pattern (behavior aimed at making the environment more beautiful), a business action pattern (exchange of goods and/or services), an education action pattern (teaching individuals), and social contact action pattern (having interpersonal relations of any kind). In the waiting room of a psychiatric clinic, one might observe some formal educational activity (perhaps a physician's assistant instructing persons regarding the use of medications), a social activity (one patient talking to another), or a some business activity (paying a bill). Barker et al. described certain "behavior mechanisms" that could be documented, such as participation (the percentage of time spent in talking) and tempo (how quickly patients move in and out of the setting). Among these "mechanisms" that the observers recorded were affective behavior (overt expressions of emotionality), talking, and manipulation (using one's hands to reach for a magazine, for instance).

Like other single-case studies, ecologic psychological studies are open to obvious criticisms. If the investigator is a "participant observer," then he/she potentially biases the situation by actively interacting with the environment that is to be objectively described. Goffman assumed the role of assistant to the athletic director, and, when pressed, avowed himself to be a student of recreation and community life: He purposefully misled the staff and therefore could not truly maintain "natural" contact with the staff, as if he were only an assistant to the athletic director.

At times ecologic psychologic studies involve the simple subjective recording of one's experience (as Goffman did). More often, however, observers (like those described in the Barker study) use formal methods to record the events they witness. Such recording requires the use of scales, and the reliability and validity of these scales (see Chapter 10) must be established.

Finally, it is unclear to what extent one can generalize from such studies. Goffman, for instance, studied only a single institution, St. Elizabeth's Hospital in Washington, DC. Though when he performed the fieldwork, during the mid-1950s, there were striking similarities across many state-run mental hospitals throughout the United States, each had unique characteristics. St. Elizabeth's Hospital was much larger than many such hospitals, it was a federal rather than a state institution, and it had been used by the National Institute of Mental Health as a place to study mental disorders. Thus, it was not typical of a state mental hospital in, for example, Nebraska or California. Such studies do provide insight into the interactions of persons with their environment as well as clues for developing hypotheses that can later be tested by using more objective methods.

Problem Set

Blazer (1996) reported the case of a 77-year-old man who experienced a severe episode of major depression and was treated with electroconvulsive therapy. The case presentation was interdigitated with the author's commentary on "the long road to recovery" after treatment with electroconvulsive therapy and supportive psychotherapy for 18 months following diagnosis. Though symptoms such as sleep and appetite disturbance responded quickly to treatment, the patient and family did not believe he had recovered until 18 months after the treatment was initiated. When the patient began to play golf again, on a regular basis, the family was convinced he had recovered. He noted that "this case illustrates two critical issues related to the course and management of severe major depressive episodes in late life." First, the typical dichotomous approach to describing the course of major depression (recovery/ relapse) does not capture the richness and complexity of recovery as well as the time it takes to recover following an episode of major depression. Second, if such a patient became "lost" in a managed care environment where careful monitoring over time by a person skilled in working with severe depressive disorders is not possible, quality of care for such a patient would be compromised.

Questions

1. What was the educational aim of this case?

2. To what extent can a clinical investigator generalize from this case, such as generalizing the time to recovery following a severe episode of major depression?

3. Can this case presentation be used to critique the health care system?

Answers

1. This case educates as a "prototypical example" (Neale and Liebert, 1973) of a severe major depressive episode in an older adult. The author suggested that the recovery from a severe episode requires a longer period of time than is typically given in textbooks and describes a case where the symptoms typically monitored by depression rating scales return to near baseline relatively soon after treatment was initiated, yet neither the patient nor the family endorsed "recovery" until many months afterward.

2. This case is suggestive but the reader should not be quick to generalize. The author suggested that typical rating scales, such as the global rating scale of functioning embedded in *DSM-IV* or the Hamilton Rating Scale for Depression, should be complemented with more qualitative assessments attuned to the patient's perceptions in order to best "track recovery from an episode." Perhaps the development of a complementary scale or a set of questions that could capture the quality of the patient's experience might be stimulated by this case.

3. The author did what many investigators and clinicians do when they either encounter a bad experience with new forms of health care delivery or recognize the value of an old form of health care delivery (in this case the psychiatrist continuing to see the patient well after usual managed care practice would encourage referral back to a primary care physician). Namely, they tend to generalize based on their experience with the new form or their sense of the old form's. Yet a system of health care delivery like managed care cannot be evaluated from the presentation of a single case. Psychiatrists and other mental care providers face major challenges with new health systems. It is all too tempting to use case reports (either positive or negative) to plead the case that the system does (or does not) provide for adequate treatment of the mentally ill. Case reports can illustrate potential weaknesses in the system which can be evaluated by more objective methods, such as comparative studies of recovery and satisfaction with care between treated depressed patients randomized to follow-up by psychiatrists and primary care physicians.

REFERENCES

Barker R.G. 1968. *Ecological Psychology: Concepts and Methods for Studying the Environment of Human Behavior*. Stanford CA: Stanford University Press.

Blazer D.G. 1996. Severe episode of depression in late life: the long road to recovery. *American Journal of Psychiatry* 153: 620–623.

Blazer D.G., Haller L. 1975. Pentazocine psychosis: a case of persistent delusion. *Disease of the Nervous System* 36: 404–440.

Goffman E. 1961. *Asylums: Essays on the Social Situation of Mental Patients and Other Inmates*. New York: Anchor Books.

Goffman J.M., McFall R.M. 1972. Self-monitoring effects in a program for potential high school dropouts: a time series analysis, *Journal of Consulting and Clinical Psychology* 39: 273–281.

Klerman G.L., Weissman M.M., Rounsaville B.J., Chevron E.S. 1984. *Interpersonal Psychotherapy of Depression*. New York: Basic Books.

Neale J.M., Liebert R.M. 1973. *Science and Behavior: An Introduction to Methods of Research*. Englewood Cliffs: Prentice Hall.

Physicians' Desk Reference (48th ed.). 1994. Montvale, Medical Economics Data, p. 2121.

Schneider K. 1959. *Clinical Psychopathology*. Translated by Hamilton M.W., Anderson E.W. New York: Gruene and Statton.

Sobel W., Wolski R., Cancro R., Makari G.J. 1996. Interpersonal relatedness and paranoid schizophrenia. *American Journal of Psychiatry* 153: 1084–1087.

Twemblow S.W., Warnock J.K. 1977. Single-subject methodology: case history and time-series design, In *A Clinician's Guide to Research Design* (ed. Goldstein G.), pp. 239–255. Chicago: Nelson-Hall.

Volkow N.D., Wang G.J., Gatley S.J., Fowler J.S., Ding Y.S., Logan J., Hitzmann R., Angrist B., Lieberman J. 1996. Temporal relationship between the pharmacokinetics of methylphenidate in the human brain and its behavioral and cardiovascular effects. *Psychopharmacology* 123: 26–33.

5

DESCRIPTIVE STUDIES

OBJECTIVES

- To distinguish a descriptive study from an analytic study.
- To describe common sources of data used in descriptive studies.
- To identify the four kinds of descriptive epidemiologic studies and their advantages and disadvantages.
- To interpret measures of frequency in descriptive studies.
- To recognize how descriptive studies can be used for analytic studies of association.

CASE EXAMPLE

Combining data from three national surveys, Escobedo and Peddicord (1996) examined smoking prevalence in successive U.S. birth cohorts by gender, race, and education ($n = 112,090$). Among white female high school graduates, peak smoking prevalence increased in the first three successive birth cohorts beginning with the group born between 1908 and 1917; then it leveled off and decreased slightly in later cohorts. Among white women without a high school education, however, peak smoking prevalence continued to increase in each successive cohort (28%, 43%, 52%, 55%, 65%, and 71%, respectively), and peak prevalence appears to have occurred at progressively younger ages for each cohort (Figure 5–1).

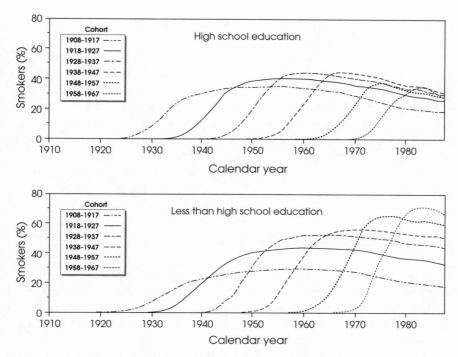

FIGURE 5–1. Smoking prevalence among birth cohorts of U.S. white women with and without a high school education (adapted from Escobedo and Peddicord, 1996).

INTRODUCTION

Nicotine dependence is one of several Axis-I nicotine-related disorders included in *DSM-III-R* (1987), and *DSM-IV* (1994). The disorder characterizes 50–80% of U.S. smokers, 85% of whom express a desire to stop smoking and 5% of whom succeed unaided each year (*DSM-IV*, 1994). The population distribution of psychiatric disorders and related behaviors, such as cigarette smoking, is often traced by using a *descriptive study.* Descriptive studies are performed when relatively little is known about the distribution, natural history, or risk factors for a disorder. A descriptive study provides a measure of the frequency or trends over time of a disorder in a population or community so that specific etiologic hypotheses can be generated. *Analytic studies*, on the other hand, are conducted to test hypotheses about risk factors, the magnitude of their effects, or interventions targeted at them (Kleinbaum et al., 1982).

The classical features of descriptive studies of disorders involve clinical features of a disorder, time, place, person, and changes over time. Descriptive studies answer the questions: Who has the disorder? Where are the rates of the disorder highest and lowest? Is the disorder common or rare? Does the prevalence of the disorder change over time?

In the example of smoking prevalence, the authors' objective was to assess long-term trends in cigarette smoking in gender and education subgroups. Using several surveys, Escobedo and Peddicord (1996) first estimated the percentage of the U.S. population that had ever smoked cigarettes, the age at which they began smoking cigarettes, and, among former smokers, how long it had been since they last smoked regularly. Next they estimated the prevalence rate of cigarette smoking among U.S. adults in each year between 1908 and 1967 separately by subgroups of the population: men and women; whites, African-Americans, and Hispanic Americans; and according to when the individual was born (*birth cohort*).

DATA SOURCES FOR DESCRIPTIVE STUDIES

Descriptive studies often depend on data that are routinely collected and widely available, making such research particularly accessible to new investigators and public health workers. Other descriptive studies are undertaken purposefully, such as the U.S. National Comorbidity Study (Kessler et al., 1994) and the Edmonton (Canada) Survey of Psychiatric Disorders (Orn et al., 1988).

Sources of data for descriptive studies are listed in Table 5–1. *Census data*, collected by most nations periodically (usually at 10-year intervals), are conventionally based on simultaneous individual enumeration of all persons within a defined territory (Nam, 1994). Census data can be used to describe the distribution of a

TABLE 5–1. Common sources of descriptive data

- National censuses (periodic reporting)
- Civil registration systems (continuous reporting)
    Annual series of vital statistics
    Mortality registries
- Population registers
- Case registers
    National
    Regional/local
- Hospital or clinic admission and discharge statistics
- Population-based national health surveys
- Sample surveys of psychiatric disorders
    International surveys
    National surveys
    Multiple community surveys
    Regional/local surveys

population by characteristics such as age, gender, racial/ethnic composition, income, urban–rural residence, and type of dwelling (e.g., U.S. Bureau of the Census, 1990) at a single well-defined point in time.

Vital statistics, in contrast, are compiled on a continuous basis by civil registration systems responsible for maintaining complete legal records of births, deaths, marriages, divorces, adoptions, and other changes in civil status of individuals. Data collected locally or regionally are forwarded regularly to central agencies such as the U.S. National Center for Health Statistics (Kovar, 1989; U.S. National Center for Health Statistics, 1995) and the Australian Bureau of Statistics (Jorm et al., 1989). Where coverage by the civil registration system is incomplete, systematic sample surveys, such as India's Sample Registration System (Padmanabha, 1984), may be used to generate more accurate series of birth and death statistics.

Annual series of vital statistics can be used to examine trends such as the increased frequency of suicide since 1980 among elderly white U.S. males, illustrated in Figure 5–2 (U.S. National Center for Health Statistics, 1985–1994). The ongoing series of reports by the Centers for Disease Control provide additional in-

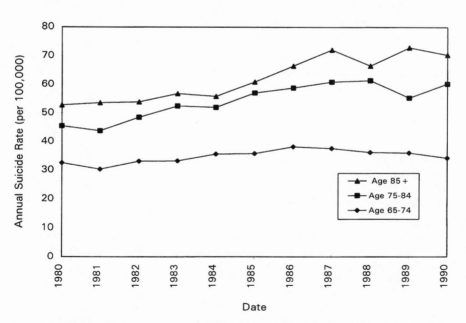

Suicide Rates in Elderly White Males, 1980-1990

FIGURE 5–2. Suicide rates in elderly white males, 1980–1990. Data from U.S. National Center for Health Statistics, 1985–1994 (annual). *Vital Statistics of the United States, 1980–1990. Vol. II: Mortality, Part A.*

formation on morbidity and mortality (U.S. Centers for Disease Control and Prevention, 1995).

Investigators may also link vital statistics to respondent data gathered from other sources. Such a procedure requires linking variables common to both sources, such as name and official identification number. In the United States, the National Death Index (NDI) is a valuable resource for record linkage (Bilgrad, 1995). The NDI lists cause of death, place of death, and other data commonly found on death certificates according to social security number, name, birth date, address, and other characteristics. In a few nations (e.g., Denmark and the Netherlands) community registrars link the records generated by the civil registration system for each individual with other records to form an integrated body of data known as a *population register* (Nam, 1994).

Psychiatric case registers are systematic compilations of data representing all individuals identified with psychiatric disorders who either (1) live within a delimited geographic area or (2) seek treatment at a medical institution which maintains a registry (Mortensen, 1995). Case register data represent a valuable source of information for descriptive studies of the incidence and prevalence of psychiatric disorders, particularly in Scandinavia and Israel, in which comprehensive psychiatric registers are maintained for national populations. Psychiatric registers are maintained at the regional or local level in a number of nations which have no centralized registry. Examples of psychiatric case registers are listed in Table 5–2. Case registers for a medical disorder can only be as complete as the proportion of affected persons with that disorder who come to the attention of a reporting clinician. Accordingly, even the most meticulously maintained psychiatric case registers may underrepresent those disorders which are not dependably associated with help-seeking behavior.

TABLE 5–2. Examples of psychiatric case registers

National:
  Denmark: Psychiatric Central Register (Munk-Jorgensen et al., 1993)
  Israel: Psychiatric Case Register (Lerner, 1992)
  Norway: Central Register for Severe Mental Disorders (Saugstad and Odegard, 1986)
  Sweden: Psychiatric Case Register (Allgulander, 1994)

Regional/Local:
  Australia (Victoria state): Victoria Psychiatric Case Register (Herrman et al., 1994)
  Germany, Mannheim: Cumulative Psychiatric Case Register (Weyerer and Hafner, 1989)
  Italy, Verona: South Verona Psychiatric Case Register (Tansella et al., 1993)
  Japan, Nagasaki: Nagasaki Mental Health Centre registry (Gulbinat et al., 1992)
  Netherlands, Groningen: Groningen Psychiatric Case Register (Sytema, 1991)
  U.K. (England), London: Camberwell Psychiatric Case Register (Der and Bebbington, 1987)
  United States, (NY state): Monroe County Psychiatric Register (Lehman et al., 1984)

Hospital admission and discharge statistics represent an alternative source of information for descriptive studies in nations or regions for which case register data are unavailable. Centrally compiled statistics in some nations (e.g., Canada) include data on admission, length of stay, and discharge for psychiatric or mental hospitals and the psychiatric units of general hospitals (U.S. National Center for Health Statistics, 1994). In the U.S., the National Institute of Mental Health compiles statistics on hospital admissions and discharges associated with psychiatric conditions, and the Center for Mental Health Services collects data from private psychiatrists and inpatient and outpatient mental health centers at the state or county level (U.S. Center for Mental Health Services, 1994).

Prevalence rates for psychiatric disorders are primarily based on broad-based surveys. Periodic population-based national surveys of general health often include information on psychiatric conditions. Descriptive profiles of such studies are available for a number of nations in the *International Health Data Reference Guide* (U.S. National Center for Health Statistics, 1994). In addition, sample surveys focused specifically on psychiatric disorders have been conducted at a variety of scales ranging from collaborative multinational efforts to national, regional, and local surveys; examples are listed in Table 5–3.

An alternative to the national survey is the *multiple community survey*, such as the U.S. Epidemiologic Catchment Area (ECA) Survey (Leaf et al., 1991; Chapter 6). During the early 1980s, approximately 19,000 community residents of Baltimore, New Haven, North Carolina, St. Louis, and Los Angeles were interviewed using the Diagnostic Interview Schedule (DIS) developed for the U.S. National Institute of Mental Health (Robins and Regier, 1991). Follow-up interviews were conducted a year later to provide information on incidence, remission, and recurrence of psychiatric disorders. Communities selected for such surveys are usually chosen to generate a sample which is as representative as possible of the diversity of the national population to which investigators wish to generalize their findings.

The case example of time trends in smoking behaviors included data taken from both national and multiple community surveys of general health. Data on white and African-American subjects were collected as part of the National Health Interview Survey (NHIS), a primary source of information on the health of U.S. civilians (Benson and Marano, 1994). The NHIS, periodically conducted using a stratified sample of U.S. households, was administered to adults 18 years of age and older (Kovar and Poe, 1985; Massey et al., 1989). Data on Hispanic-American subjects in the case example were gathered as part of a multiple community survey, the Hispanic Health and Nutrition Examination Survey (HHANES), also administered to adults 18 years of age and older. The HHANES included a stratified probability sample of residents from three geographic areas representing the majority of the U.S. Hispanic population: Mexican Americans living in five southwestern states (Arizona, California, Colorado, New Mexico, and Texas), Puerto Rican Americans

TABLE 5–3. Examples of sample surveys of psychiatric disorders

- International surveys
    WHO Collaborative Study (Colombia, India, Philippines, Sudan):
    Frequency of childhood mental disorders in primary health care, total $n = 925$
    (Giel et al., 1981)
    Cross National Collaborative Group on Obsessive Compulsive Disorder (Canada,
    Germany, Korea, New Zealand, Puerto Rico, Taiwan, U. S.):
    Epidemiology of obsessive compulsive disorder, total $n = 41,425$ (Weissman et al.,
    1994)
    Nigeria and U.S.: Prevalence of Alzheimer's disease/dementia in African and
    African-American elders, $n = 2,494$ in Ibadan, Nigeria, and $n = 2,318$ in
    Indianapolis, U. S. (Hendrie et al., 1995)

- National surveys
    Greece: Nationwide psychiatric case identification study, $n = 4,292$ (Madianos and
    Stefanos, 1992)
    Kenya: Nationwide survey on prevalence of mental disorders, $n = 881$ (Dhadpale
    et al., 1989)
    New Zealand: National survey of elders with mental retardation, $n = 1,063$ (Hand,
    1993)
    U. K.: National Survey of Psychiatric Morbidity, $n = 10,000$ (Jenkins and Meltzer,
    1995)
    U. S.: National Comorbidity Survey, $n = 8,098$ (Kessler et al., 1994; Blazer et al.,
    1994)

- Multiple community surveys
    Tanzania, Morogoro and Moshi regions: National Mental Health Programme pilot
    tests, $n = 5,681$ (Schulsinger and Jablensky, 1991)
    Taiwan, 4 urban and 4 rural communities: Survey of dementia in elders, $n = 5,297$
    (Liu et al., 1995)
    U. S., 5 communities: Epidemiologic Catchment Area survey, $n = 19,182$ (Robins
    and Regier, 1991)

- Regional/local surveys
    Belarus, Gomel region: Postdisaster survey of mental health problems, $n = 1,617$
    (Havenaar et al., 1996)
    Brazil, Sao Paulo: Survey of psychotropic use, $n = 1,742$ (Mari et al., 1993)
    Canada, Edmonton: Edmonton Survey of Psychiatric Disorders, $n = 3,258$ (Orn
    et al., 1988)
    China, Shanghai: Shanghai Survey of Alzheimer's Disease and Dementia, $n = 5,055$
    (Zhang et al., 1990)
    Dubai: Dubai Community Psychiatric Survey of women, $n = 300$ (Ghubash et al.,
    1992)
    Hong Kong: Shatin Community Mental Health Survey, $n = 7,229$ (Chen et al., 1993)
    India, Kerala state: Epidemiology of dementia, $n = 2,067$ (Shaji et al., 1996)
    Italy, Florence: Community survey of mood disorders, $n = 1,000$ (Faravelli et al.,
    1990)
    Lesotho, "Midvill" village: Community prevalence of depression and anxiety,
    $n = 356$ (Hollifield et al., 1990)

(continued)

TABLE 5–3. *(Continued)*

Korea, Seoul: Lifetime prevalence of mental illness, $n = 3,134$ (Lee et al., 1990)

Malaysia: Prevalence survey of mental disorders among children, $n = 507$ (Kasmini et al., 1993)

New Zealand: Christchurch Psychiatric Epidemiology Study, $n = 1,498$ (Wells et al., 1989)

Spain, Zaragoza: Prevalence of dementia and depression in elderly, $n = 1,080$ (Lobo et al., 1995)

U.K. (England), London: Guy's Age Concern Survey of physical health and psychiatric disorder, $n = 890$ (Lindesay, 1990)

living in New York City, and Cuban Americans living in Dade County, FL (U.S. National Center for Health Statistics, 1985).

TYPES OF DESCRIPTIVE STUDIES

There are four basic types of descriptive epidemiologic studies: ecologic studies, case reports and series, cross-sectional surveys, and temporal analyses (Table 5–4). *Ecologic studies* have as their unit of analysis some aggregate of individuals, such as residents of a geographic area or members of a cohort living during a particular time frame. This approach to the study of disorders differs from most epidemiologic designs, which have the single individual as the unit of study. For example, an ecologic study might find a significant association between the number of vending machines in a state and the estimated prevalence of smoking behavior among young teens. Although the two variables are significantly associated at the regional level, the existence of this association does not necessarily indicate that removing cigarette vending machines will have any impact on the smoking behavior of individual teenagers. An aggregate association can occur in the absence of any cause-and-effect relationship between two variables. Perhaps the prevalences of vending machines and smoking behaviors among minors are directly dependent on one or more variables not included in the study.

The bias that can occur because an association observed between variables on an aggregate level is erroneously assumed to represent a true association on the individual level is commonly referred to as the *ecologic fallacy*. Ecologic studies cannot directly link an exposure with a disorder; nor can they distinguish between cause and effect. Furthermore, ecologic studies cannot control for the effects of potential confounding factors, as discussed in Chapter 7.

Nevertheless, ecologic studies can serve the purpose of generating hypotheses about etiologic factors associated with outcomes of public interest which can be tested using studies of individuals. Also, ecologic studies may be most appropriate where broad societal or cultural phenomena are of interest. The causal web of

TABLE 5–4. Strengths and weaknesses of descriptive studies

Ecologic studies

Strengths

- Assist in generating hypotheses
- Illustrate broad population trends
- Implicate population-level risk factors and prognostic factors

Weaknesses

- Do not directly link exposures with disorders
- Do not distinguish cause and effect
- Do not account for confounding factors

Case series

Strengths

- Assist in generating hypotheses
- Provide the opportunity for comprehensive assessment of cases

Weaknesses

- Have poor generalizability

Cross-sectional prevalence studies

Strengths

- Are less expensive than longitudinal studies
- Are broadly generalizable

Weaknesses

- Provide limited understanding of the natural history and etiology of a disease
- Cannot account for competing risks to subjects from other outcomes
- Provide limited opportunity for diagnostic assessment

Temporal analyses (historical trend studies)

Strengths

- Potential to disaggregate the effects of age, period and cohort
- Broadly generalizable

Weaknesses

- Cannot account for competing risks to participants from other outcomes, e.g., mortality
- Provide limited opportunity for diagnostic assessment, usually relying on secondary data sources, e.g., death certificates for suicide

---

disorders such as major depression requires conceptualization of the social and historical contexts, and group-level risk factors as well as individual risk factors may be amenable to change. Rose (1992) notes that even small improvements in the health of a "sick population" may be more effective than major efforts to improve the health of "sick individuals."

Case series represent a second type of descriptive studies. Case series are collections of individual *case reports* which may occur within a fairly short period of time and draw attention to an epidemic or a previously unexamined disorder. For example, during and after World War II, psychiatrists became particularly interested in acute grief reactions. Lindemann (1944) interviewed bereaved relatives of soldiers, bereaved victims of the Cocoanut Grove fire disaster, bereaved relatives of medical patients, and bereaved psychiatric patients and reported a series of case histories describing the symptoms, course, and management of normal, morbid, and anticipatory grief reactions. Other investigators have developed measurable hypotheses from these important observations and tested them in quantitative studies of the natural history and nosology of grief reactions.

The limitation of case series concerns their generalizability. Because they are based on the experience of a limited number of patients, the apparent relationships between risk factors and an outcome may be coincidental. Typically, the number of persons in a case series is too small to estimate measures of the frequency of psychiatric disorders or to calculate usable estimates of the association between risk factor and disorder. However, a case series, like an ecologic study, may help to generate hypotheses which can then be tested with study designs that include a comparison group and adequate numbers of subjects.

A third type of descriptive study is the *cross-sectional (prevalence) study*. In such a study, a sample is surveyed simultaneously for both the prevalence of a disorder and a variety of exposure factors. The survey is usually conducted within a limited time frame, such as a calendar year, and thus provides a snapshot of the distribution of a disorder (or disorders) and exposures in a circumscribed population at a specific point in time. In the example of smoking prevalence in U.S. birth cohorts, Escobedo and Peddicord (1996) used data from five cross-sectional NHIS surveys performed in 1978, 1979, 1980, 1987, and 1988 and three cross-sectional HHANES surveys from 1982–1984. Separate cross-sectional surveys were combined to increase the overall size of the sample and therefore its representativeness of the entire U.S. population. The five particular NHIS surveys selected represented the only years in which questionnaires included items about both the initiation and the cessation of smoking.

Cross-sectional studies based on routinely collected data or with checklist-style assessment methods have the advantage of being relatively inexpensive. Furthermore, they can be broadly generalizable because the samples drawn are typically from entire communities. Cross-sectional studies often provide the cases and controls used in case-control studies (Chapter 8), even if the original sampling procedures did not target a precise number of cases and controls. These secondary analyses of descriptive data are called *"nested" case-control studies*. A more detailed description of cross-sectional survey methodology is given in Chapter 6.

Cross-sectional surveys can have several limitations. First, assessment of exposures and disorders at a single point in time limits the understanding of the chronology of cause and effect. This was not so much a problem in the smoking study (Escobedo and Peddicord, 1996), in which gender, race, and educational attainment antedate lifetime smoking behavior. But in studies where exposures may be cumulative and/or changeable through time (e.g., stressful life events), unraveling the etiologic relationship between onset of a disorder and the various exposures of interest is not possible with cross-sectional data. Longitudinal designs (Chapter 7) are needed to ascertain the temporal relationships between exposure and disease.

Another problem with cross-sectional studies is the competing risk of mortality, i.e., affected persons may be underrepresented because they were more likely to have died prior to the study for some reason related to the disorder being studied. For example, a lower proportion of smokers than nonsmokers in older cohorts might have survived to be counted in the 1988 survey, thus biasing downward the estimates of overall smoking prevalence among persons born earlier.

Finally, the determination of disorder status is likely to be less specific in community prevalence studies than in clinically based case-control studies because investigators must rely on data collection methods which do not include extensive medical evaluations of the disorder. When a national or regional descriptive study includes thorough diagnostic workups, such as the National Comorbidity Study, it is neither cheap nor quick to perform. Clinicians may find descriptive studies easier to mount in smaller, more circumscribed communities, as is the case in the problem set following this chapter.

The fourth type of descriptive study is the *temporal analysis* or *historical trend* study. Historical trends refer to changes that occur gradually over long periods of time, usually several decades. For example, Blazer's (1991) analysis of historical trends in suicide showed that the prevalence of suicides dropped across successive cohorts of U.S. men. Among 60-year-old white men born in 1902, 1912, and 1922, suicide rates were respectively 39, 34, and 27 per 100,000. The study of Escobedo and Peddicord (1996) documented historical trends in smoking prevalence: peak prevalence rose from 28% to 71% across cohorts of women without a high school diploma and occurred at progressively younger ages in each cohort (Figure 5–1). Evaluating a historical trend in prevalence of a disorder requires the investigator to consider the age of the subject, the (calendar) time at which the data were collected, and the birth cohort to which the individual belongs, any of which may be associated with having the disorder. Effects of any of the above (*age, period*, or *cohort*) which appear in a descriptive study to be associated with the prevalence of a disorder can be tested subsequently using an analytic study. Age, period, and cohort are discussed in more detail in Chapter 7.

DESCRIPTIVE MEASURES

The most common measure used in a descriptive study of a disorder is prevalence. Calculation of prevalence is described in Chapter 3. Annual mortality rates, or rates of other (nondeath) events that occur during a circumscribed time (e.g., 1-year institutionalization rates) are also typical measures calculated from descriptive data. State phenomena measured on a continuum (e.g., the severity of depressive symptoms or the size of a patient's social network) are often assessed in descriptive studies and presented in terms of their range of values or the average value in the sample. These latter measures are commonly employed in descriptive studies and are described more fully in Chapter 12.

Problem Set

In 1982, John Kane and colleagues noted both the efficacy of neuroleptic treatment for long-term management of schizophrenia and also the growing concern over a concurrent increased prevalence of tardive dyskinesia (TD) among treated patients. In 56 studies of neuroleptic-treated patients ($n = 34,555$), the average prevalence of TD was 20%. In 19 studies of untreated (psychiatric and nonpsychiatric) samples ($n = 10,944$), the average prevalence of TD was 5%, but the range of reported prevalence rates among untreated patients was 0–36.7%.

The authors speculated that either psychiatric or neurologic comorbidity or age might be responsible for the variability in these estimates across samples. They undertook a small descriptive study of the prevalence of abnormal involuntary movements in a non-clinical sample of elderly volunteers ($n = 150$) from a senior citizen's center (Kane et al., 1982). Respondents were rated on the Simpson Dyskinesia Scale (Simpson et al., 1979), modified to include a global rating of severity (range: 0–6), and were screened for a current or past history of psychiatric or neurological condition (e.g., stroke, Parkinson's, epilepsy) or treatment. Characteristics of their sample are presented in Table 5–5.

Questions

After examining Table 5–5, answer the following questions:

1. Describe the person, place, and time parameters of this study.

2. What is the definition and prevalence of "normal" elderly in this sample? In what ways may this sample represent or fail to represent all "normal" elderly? What is the prevalence of mild and moderate involuntary movements among "normal" older persons?

TABLE 5–5. Prevalence of abnormal involuntary movements in elderly volunteers

	GROUP I NORMAL	GROUP II NEUROLOGICAL HISTORY	GROUP III PSYCHIATRIC HISTORY
N	127	17	6
Males	53	5	0
Females	74	12	6
Mean age	72.5 (± 7.3)	71.3 (± 5.1)	72.5 (± 7.3)
Global rating questionable	8% (10/127)	12% (2/17)	0
Global rating mild	4% (5/127)	6% (1/17)	0
Global rating moderate	0	0	17% (1/6)

Data from Kane et al., 1982

3. What is the prevalence of neurological and psychiatric comorbidity in this sample of elderly? How representative of these two types of patients are the two study groups? What is the prevalence of TD among older persons who have neurological and psychiatric comorbidity?

4. Between which comparison groups do differences appear to exist?

5. In what ways might a knowledge of the prevalence estimates reported for mild symptoms among "normal" elders enhance your ability to conduct an analytic study of the etiology of TD?

Answers

1. The respondents were older American men and women who were independent enough to attend a senior citizens' center in the early 1980s. Their race, socioeconomic status, education, and family medical history are not known.

2. Approximately 85% of the sample was "normal," i.e., reporting no past history of a psychiatric or neurological disorder or treatment for these conditions. This sample may be underrepresentative of frail elders who are unable to attend a senior citizens' center for other reasons besides neurological or psychiatric incapacity. It may also underrepresent healthier elders whose families and social resources are plentiful and who do not choose to attend a center. The 4–8% prevalence ratings for mild–questionable involuntary movements are consonant with the average prevalence rates from untreated samples (5%) but fall within the lower range of published values (0–36.7%).

3. Approximately 11% of the sample reported neurological conditions, treatments, or medications. About 4% reported psychiatric conditions, treatments, or medications. These two groups were extremely small and so likely do not represent the variety of neurological and psychiatric conditions and treatments potentially associated with involuntary movements, particularly the more severe and debilitating neurological and psychiatric conditions and courses.

4. The 6–12% prevalence rate of involuntary movements among neurologic patients is only slightly higher than the average published prevalence rates of untreated samples and is therefore likely not different from the rates among "normal" elders in this study. The 17% prevalence rate of moderate involuntary movements among psychiatric patients is closer to the 20% average prevalence among neuroleptic-treated patient samples. This suggests that studies of untreated samples with high TD prevalence rates may indeed have been confounded by persons with comorbidity associated with TD.

5. Baseline rates of a disorder in a population serve as a benchmark for comparing groups who are exposed and unexposed to a putative risk factor. One would expect to see a similar 4–5% prevalence rate of TD across groups who differed only on a given exposure if that exposure were, in fact, unrelated to TD.

REFERENCES

Allgulander C. 1994. Suicide and mortality patterns in anxiety neurosis and depressive neurosis. *Archives of General Psychiatry* 51: 708–712.

Benson V., Marano, M.A. 1994. Current estimates from the National Health Interview Survey, United States, 1993. National Center for Health Statistics *Vital and Health Statistics* 10(190). Washington, DC: U.S. Government Printing Office.

Bilgrad R. 1995. *National Death Index User's Manual*. (revised ed.). DHHS Pub. No. (PHS) 95–0125-P. Hyattsville, MD: Public Health Service.

Blazer D.G. 1991. Suicide risk factors in the elderly: an epidemiological study. *Journal of Geriatric Psychiatry* 24: 175–190.

Blazer D.G., Kessler R.C., McGonagle K.A., Swartz M.S. 1994. The prevalence and distribution of major depression in a national community sample: the National Comorbidity Survey. *American Journal of Psychiatry* 151: 979–986.

Chen C.N., Wong J., Lee N., Chan-ho, M.W., Lau J.T., Fung M. 1993. The Shatin Community Mental Health Survey in Hong Kong: II. Major findings. *Archives of General Psychiatry* 50: 125–133.

Der G., Bebbington P. 1987. Depression in inner London: a register study. *Social Psychiatry* 22: 73–84.

Dhadpale M., Cooper G., Cartwright-Taylor L. 1989. Prevalence and presentation of depressive illness in a primary health care setting in Kenya. *American Journal of Psychiatry* 146: 659–661.

DSM-III-R. 1987. *Diagnostic and Statistical Manual of Mental Disorders: DSM-III-R,* 3rd ed., revised. Washington, DC: American Psychiatric Association.

DSM-IV. 1994. *Diagnostic and Statistical Manual of Mental Disorders: DSM-IV,* 4th ed. Washington, DC: American Psychiatric Association.

Escobedo L.G., Peddicord J.P. 1996. Smoking prevalence in U.S. birth cohorts: the influence of gender and education. *American Journal of Public Health* 86: 231–236.

Faravelli C., Degl'Innocenti B.G., Benedetta G., Aiazzi L., Incerpi G., Pallanti S. 1990. Epidemiology of mood disorders: a community survey in Florence. *Journal of Affective Disorders* 20: 135–141.

Ghubash R., Hamdi E., Bebbington P. 1992. The Dubai Community Psychiatric Survey: I. Prevalence and socio-demographic correlates. *Social Psychiatry and Psychiatric Epidemiology* 27: 53–61.

Giel R., de Arango M.V., Climent C.E., Harding T.W., Ibrahim H.H., Ladrido-Ignacio L., Murthy R.S., Salazar M.C., Wig N.N., Younis Y.O. 1981. Childhood mental disorders in primary health care: results of observations in four developing countries. A report from the WHO Collaborative Study on Strategies for Extending Mental Health Care. *Pediatrics* 68: 677–683.

Gulbinat W., Dupont A., Jablensky A., Jensen O.M., Marsella A., Nakane Y., Sartorius N. 1992. Cancer incidence in schizophrenic patients: results of record linkage studies in three countries. *British Journal of Psychiatry* 161 (*Suppl.* 18): 75–85.

Hand J.E. 1993. Summary of national survey of older people with mental retardation in New Zealand. *Mental Retardation* 31: 424–428.

Havenaar J.M., van den Brink W., van den Bout J., Kasyanenko A.P., Poelijoe N.W., Wohlfarth T., Meijleriljina L.I. 1996. Mental health problems in the Gomel region (Belarus): an analysis of risk factors in an area affected by the Chernobyl disaster. *Psychological Medicine* 26: 845–855.

Hendrie H.C., Osuntokun B.O., Hall K.S., Ogunniyi A.O., Hui S.L., Unverzagt F.W., Gureje O., Rodenberg C.A., Baiyewu O., Musick B.S., Adeyinka A., Farlow M.R., Oluwole S.O., Class A., Komolafe O., Brashear A., Burdine V. 1995. Prevalence of Alzheimer's disease and dementia in two communities: Nigerian Africans and African Americans. *American Journal of Psychiatry* 152: 1485–1492.

Herrman H., Mills J., Doidge G., McGorry P., Singh B. 1994. The use of psychiatric services before imprisonment: a survey and case register linkage of sentenced prisoners in Melbourne. *Psychological Medicine* 24: 63–68.

Hollifield M., Katon W., Spain D., Pule L. 1990. Anxiety and depression in a village in Lesotho, Africa: a comparison with the United States. *British Journal of Psychiatry* 156: 343–350.

Jenkins R., Meltzer H. 1995. The national survey of psychiatric morbidity in Great Britain. *Social Psychiatry and Psychiatric Epidemiology* 30:1–4.

Jorm A.F., Henderson A.S., Jacomb P.A. 1989. Regional differences in mortality from dementia in Australia: an analysis of death certificate data. *Acta Psychiatrica Scandinavica* 79: 179–185.

Kane J.M., Weinhold P., Kinon B., Wegner J., Leader M. 1982. Prevalence of abnormal involuntary movements ("spontaneous dyskinesias") in the normal elderly. *Psychopharmacology* 77: 105–108.

Kasmini K., Kyaw O., Krishnaswamy S., Ramli H., Hassan S. 1993. A prevalence survey of mental disorders among children in a rural Malaysian village. *Acta Psychiatrica Scandinavica* 87: 253–257.

Kessler R.C., McGonagle K.A., Zhao S., Nelson C.B., Hughes M., Eshleman S., Wittchen H.-U., Kendler K.S. 1994. Lifetime and 12-month prevalence of DSM-III-R psychiatric disorders in the United States: results from the National Comorbidity Survey. *Archives of General Psychiatry* 51: 8–19.

Kleinbaum D.G., Kupper L.L., Morgenstern H. 1982. *Epidemiologic Research: Principles and Quantitative Methods.* New York: Van Nostrand Reinhold.

Kovar M.G. 1989. Data systems of the National Center for Health Statistics through the 1980's. National Center for Health Statistics *Vital and Health Statistics* 1(23). Washington, DC: U.S. Government Printing Office.

Kovar M.G., Poe G.S. 1985. The National Health Interview Survey: design 1973–84 and procedures 1975–83. National Center for Health Statistics *Vital and Health Statistics* 1(18). Washington, DC: U.S. Government Printing Office.

Leaf P.J., Myers J.K., McEvoy L.T. 1991. Procedures used in the Epidemiologic Catchment Area Study. In *Psychiatric Disorders in America: The Epidemiologic Catchment Area Study* (eds. Robins L. N., Regier D.A.), pp. 11–32. New York: Free Press.

Lee C.K., Kwak Y.S., Yamamoto J., Rhee H., Kim Y.S., Han J.H., Choi J.O., Lee Y.H. 1990. Psychiatric epidemiology in Korea: I. Gender and age differences in Seoul. *Journal of Nervous and Mental Disease* 178: 242–246.

Lehman A.F., Babigian B.M., Reed S.K. 1984. The epidemiology of treatment for chronic and nonchronic mental disorders. *Journal of Nervous and Mental Disease* 172: 658–666.

Lerner Y. 1992. Psychiatric epidemiology in Israel. *Israel Journal of Psychiatry and Related Sciences* 29: 218–228.

Lindemann E. 1944. Symptomatology and management of acute grief. *American Journal of Psychiatry* 101: 141–148.

Lindesay J. 1990. The Guy's/Age Concern Survey: physical health and psychiatric disorder in an urban elderly community. *International Journal of Geriatric Psychiatry* 5: 171–178.

Liu H.C., Lin K.N., Teng E.L., Wang S.J., Fuh J.L., Guo N.W., Chou P., Hu H.H., Chiang B.N. 1995. Prevalence and subtypes of dementia in Taiwan: a community survey of 5297 individuals. *Journal of the American Geriatrics Society* 43: 144–149.

Lobo A., Saz P., Marcos G., Dia J.-L., De la Camara C. 1995. The prevalence of dementia and depression in the elderly community in a southern European population: the Zaragoza study. *Archives of General Psychiatry* 52: 497–506.

Madianos M.G., Stefanos C.N. 1992. Who needs treatment? A nationwide psychiatric case identification study. *Psychopathology* 25: 212–217.

Mari J.J., Almeida-Filho N., Coutinho E., Andreoli S.B., Miranda C.T., Streiner D. 1993. The epidemiology of psychotropic use in the city of Sao Paulo. *Psychological Medicine* 23: 467–474.

Massey J.T., Moore T.F., Parsons V.S., Tadros W. 1989. Design and estimation for the National Health Interview Survey, 1985–94. National Center for Health Statistics *Vital and Health Statistics* 2(110). Washington, DC: U.S. Government Printing Office.

Mortensen P.B. 1995. The untapped potential of case registers and record-linkage studies in psychiatric epidemiology. *Epidemiologic Reviews* 17: 205–209.

Munk-Jorgensen P., Kastrup M., Mortensen P.B. 1993. The Danish psychiatric register as a tool in epidemiology. *Acta Psychiatrica Scandinavica* 87, (*Suppl.* 370): 27–32.

Nam, C.B. 1994. *Understanding Population Change*. Itasca, IL: F.E. Peacock.

Orn H., Newman S.C., Bland R.C. 1988. Design and field methods of the Edmonton survey of psychiatric disorders. *Acta Psychiatrica Scandinavica* 77 (*Suppl.* 338): 17–23.

Padmanabha P. 1984. Use of sample registration systems for studying levels, trends and differentials in mortality: the experience of India. In *Data Bases for Mortality Measurement*, pp. 54–65. United Nations Department of International Economic and Social Affairs, Population Studies, No. 84. (ST/ESA/SER.A/84).

Robins L.N., Regier D.A. (eds.). 1991. *Psychiatric Disorders in America: The Epidemiologic Catchment Area Study*. New York: Free Press.

Rose G. 1992. *The Strategy of Preventive Medicine*. Oxford: Oxford University Press.

Saugstad L., Odegard O. 1986. Huntington's chorea in Norway. *Psychological Medicine* 16: 39–48.

Schulsinger F., Jablensky A. (eds.). 1991. The national mental health programme in the United Republic of Tanzania: a report from WHO and DANIDA. *Acta Psychiatrica Scandinavica* 83, (*Suppl.* 364): 1–132.

Shaji S., Promodu K., Abraham T., Roy K.J., Verghese A. 1996. An epidemiological study of dementia in a rural community in Kerala, India. *British Journal of Psychiatry* 168: 745–749.

Simpson G.M., Lee H.J., Zoubak B., Gardos G.L. 1979. A rating scale for tardive dyskinesia. *Psychopharmacology* 64: 171–179.

Sytema S. 1991. Social indicators and psychiatric admission rates: a case register study in the Netherlands. *Psychological Medicine* 21: 177–184.

Tansella M., Bisoffi G., Thornicroft G. 1993. Are social deprivation and psychiatric service utilisation associated with neurotic disorders? A case register study in South Verona. *Social Psychiatry and Psychiatric Epidemiology* 28: 225–230.

U.S. Bureau of the Census. 1990. *1990 Census of Population, General Population Characteristics*. Series 1990-CP-1. Washington, DC: U.S. Bureau of the Census.

U.S. Center for Mental Health Services. 1994. *Mental Health, United States, 1994*, (eds. Mandelscheid R. W., Sonnenschein M. A.) DHHS Pub. No. (SMA) 94–3000. Washington, DC: U.S. Government Printing Office.

U.S. Centers for Disease Control and Prevention. 1995. *Morbidity and Mortality Weekly*

Report, 1993–1994 (CD-ROM format). Atlanta, GA: Centers for Disease Control and Prevention.

U.S. National Center for Health Statistics. 1985. Plan and operation of the Hispanic Health and Nutrition Examination Survey, 1982–84. National Center for Health Statistics *Vital and Health Statistics* 1(19). Washington, DC: U.S. Government Printing Office.

U.S. National Center for Health Statistics. 1985–1994. *Vital Statistics of the United States. Vol. II—Mortality, Part A.* (Annual volumes for 1980–1990). Hyattsville, MD: Public Health Service.

U.S. National Center for Health Statistics. 1994. *International Health Data Reference Guide*, 1993 (6th ed). DHHS Pub. No. (PHS) 94–1007. Washington, DC: U.S. Government Printing Office.

U.S. National Center for Health Statistics. 1995. *National Center for Health Statistics Publications* (computer file). NCHS CD-ROM. Washington, DC: U.S. Government Printing Office.

Weissman M.M., Bland R.C., Canino G.J., Greenwald S., Hwu H-G., Lee C.K., Newman S.C., Oakley-Browne M.A., Rubio-Stipec M., Wickramaratne P.J., Wittchen H-U., Yeh E-K. 1994. The cross national epidemiology of obsessive compulsive disorder. *Journal of Clinical Psychiatry* 55(3) (*Suppl.*): 5–10.

Wells J.E., Bushnell J.A., Hornblow A.R., Joyce P.R., Oakley-Browne M.A. 1989. Christchurch Psychiatric Epidemiology Study: I. Methodology and lifetime prevalence for specific psychiatric disorders. *Australia and New Zealand Journal of Psychiatry* 23: 315–326.

Weyerer S., Hafner H. 1989. The stability of the ecological distribution of the incidence of treated mental disorders in the city of Mannheim. *Social Psychiatry and Psychiatric Epidemiology* 24: 57–62.

Zhang M., Katzman R., Salmon D., Jin H., Cai G., Wang Z., Qu G., Grant I., Yu E., Levy P., Klauber M.R., Liu W.T. 1990. The prevalence of dementia and Alzheimer's disease in Shanghai, China: impact of age, gender, and education. *Annals of Neurology* 27: 428–437.

6

COMMUNITY-BASED CROSS-SECTIONAL STUDIES

OBJECTIVES

- To delineate the purpose of community-based epidemiologic studies from that of clinical studies.
- To describe and and evaluate the development of data-collecting instruments for community-based cross-sectional epidemiologic studies.
- To describe the methods for identifying a community-based cross-sectional sample.
- To describe the process of interviewing in the community.
- To review the potential for secondary data analysis of community-based cross-sectional epidemiologic studies.

CASE EXAMPLE

During the early 1980s, the National Institute of Mental Health (NIMH) launched a comprehensive study of the prevalence of mental disorders in the United States—the Epidemiologic Catchment Area (ECA) Program based on the third edition of the *Diagnostic and Statistical Manual* (American Psychiatric Association, 1980; Robins et al., 1991). Five sites in the United States were surveyed—New Haven, Baltimore, urban St. Louis and rural areas immediately bordering the city, urban and rural North

Carolina, and selected areas of Los Angeles. Each area in the study corresponded to one or more catchment areas into which the United States had been divided during the 1960s in order to distribute psychiatric services through the Community Mental Health Center movement. The North Carolina site of the ECA Program will be described to illustrate a community-based cross-sectional design.

THE GOALS OF COMMUNITY-BASED EPIDEMIOLOGIC STUDIES

During the past 10 years, no one could read any of the major journals in psychiatry without encountering an article reporting findings from a large, community-based epidemiology study. These large studies generate data suitable for a variety of study designs, such as longitudinal and case-control studies. In their overall design, however, they are probably best categorized as descriptive studies. They provide data on the frequency and distribution of psychiatric disorders in the community. This chapter is devoted to such studies because clinicians encounter reports of them so often and because they lack direct experience with the methods used in such studies.

The Epidemiologic Catchment Area (ECA) Program was a series of large, community-based surveys designed to estimate the prevalence of specific psychiatric disorders, as defined by *DSM-III*, during the early 1980s. Most previous community-based studies in the United States were designed to estimate global impairment secondary to psychiatric illness. These included the Stirling County Study and the Mid-town Manhattan Study (though specific diagnoses were abstracted from the Stirling County data, as described in Chapter 7). The earlier studies estimated the overall prevalence of mental health impairment in both urban and rural communities to be around 20%. In contrast, the ECA investigators estimated the prevalence of specific psychiatric disorders. For example, the prevalence of major depressive disorder was estimated to be 2.4% (Regier et al., 1984; Leighton et al., 1963; Srole, 1962). The aggregate of subjects who met criteria for some *DSM-III* diagnosis was approximately 20%. The ECA study also charted the distribution of psychiatric disorders by age, gender, social class, race/ethnicity, and residence as well as a number of known risk factors for psychiatric disorders such as stressful life events and impaired social support. An additional goal was to determine the use of mental health and other health services by persons with psychiatric disorders. These comprehensive goals derived from recommendations in the President's Commission on Mental Health report, which recognized major gaps in our understanding of the epidemiology of specific psychiatric disorders in the community and of the use of mental health services (*Report to the President's Commission on Mental Health*, Vol. 1, 1978).

The data derived from the ECA study permitted many investigators to pursue more specific questions. For example, the North Carolina group explored the distribution of alcohol abuse and dependence in the North Carolina sample to determine the frequency of alcohol abuse among specific subgroups in a geographic area where abstinence from alcohol is high—the Bible Belt (Blazer et al., 1987). Because of the comprehensive collection of data in community-based epidemiologic studies, investigators have the opportunity to address a wide variety of specific and previously unanswered questions.

DESIGNING A RESEARCH INSTRUMENT

When community-based epidemiologic studies are designed, many investigators want a "piece of the action." Thus, countless questions and assessment procedures may be proposed for inclusion in a survey. For the ECA studies, a total of 17,003 interviews were done in the five sites, including 3,801 in North Carolina. Data from such a large number of subjects are not easy to obtain because of cost and logistics, especially if the subjects are representative of the community as a whole. Therefore, a major task of the investigative team is to balance the interests of multiple investigators and the capabilities of the research design to derive valuable data from residents in the community.

At least two approaches to designing a study will help to ensure that the interviewers do not obtain data that are of little value. First, the shortest scales and questionnaire items available which can reasonably be expected to obtain necessary data for a particular domain should be used. In the ECA study, for example, the North Carolina team was interested in social factors as they relate to psychiatric disorders. The team could have asked many questions to determine stressors in the social environment. Instead, the team limited the questions to a few specific stressful events, such as death of a spouse during the past year, and to the individuals' perception of the impact of these events.

Second, investigators designing a community-based epidemiologic study should, if possible, include questionnaire items and scales with proven validity and reliability in previous community-based surveys. For example, most investigators could create a series of questions which would determine the "activities of daily living" or ADL of persons. Nevertheless, there are many well-tested scales assessing ADL in the literature (Katz and Akpom, 1976; OARS, 1978). Duke investigators incorporated scales developed and tested in the OARS community study into the ECA study (OARS, 1978). Investigators should therefore select an existing scale which has proven valid and reliable in previous survey research to assess life satisfaction.

Two types of assessment in community-based studies deserve special attention: the diagnosis of psychiatric disorders and the use of medications. Rarely do clinicians perform diagnostic interviews in community-based samples in the United States. (In Europe, however, psychiatrists are frequently employed in obtaining data for diagnoses and tests of impairment (Bebbington et al., 1981; Henderson et al., 1979). The instrument most commonly used is the Present State Examination, a structured psychiatric interview. The cost of sending a clinician to the community is the reason U.S. investigators favor lay interviewers. Therefore, standardized instruments have been designed which permit the assessment of symptoms and the diagnosis of psychiatric disorders by nonclinicians. In the ECA Program, the Diagnostic Interview Schedule (DIS) was used as the standardized instrument to determine cases of psychiatric disorders and therefore served as the foundation of the entire research project (Robins et al., 1981a,b). The DIS elicited the presence or absence of a series of criterion-based symptoms for *DSM-III* diagnoses, the duration of these symptoms, and their severity. Severity was assessed in terms of whether the subject interviewed had ever sought professional help for that symptom or had taken a medication to treat the symptom. The interview takes approximately 1 hour to complete. The answers to these questions were then analyzed by a computer program which sorted these community-dwelling subjects into the cases or noncases of specific *DSM-III* diagnoses. Controversy arose regarding the reliability and validity of the DIS. (For a more general discussion of validity and reliability, see Chapter 10.) Such controversy regarding the DIS, however, accompanies virtually all diagnostic instruments administered by nonclinicians to a community sample, for these instruments are inherently limited by the lack of clinical judgment which can be applied to the diagnosis of the psychiatric disorder. One compromise is to employ a nonphysician clinician, such as a psychiatric nurse or social worker. The investigator must therefore make difficult choices regarding the standardized interview to be used and the type of interviewer to employ, for the success or failure of the entire survey depends upon the identification of clinically relevant syndromes.

A second area which proves difficult to assess in community surveys is the use of medications. Most clinicians who do not have experience with survey research assume that medication use can easily be obtained in community surveys. In fact, the use of medications is among the most difficult topics to assess accurately in the community. Persons do not know the names of the medications they are taking, nor the dose. In addition, they frequently forget medications which they take on an as-needed basis. For this reason, the best means for obtaining information regarding medication use is to ask the subject bring her or his pill bottles, both prescription and nonprescription, to the interviewer, and for the interviewer and the subject to discuss each container to determine whether the subject presently uses the medication and how frequently the medication is used. This process is time-consuming, requiring 10 minutes or more on average for older subjects, but is generally the only means by which accurate assessment of medication is possible. Even so, accurate data can usually be obtained only for the 24–48 hours prior to the interview. A week prior to the interview is frequently too long for subjects, especially older subjects, to remember which medications they are taking. In the ECA Program, the North Carolina team used colored pictures of medications, such as found in the *Physicians' Desk Reference*, to prompt individuals regarding their medication use. The increased frequency of use of generic medications during the 1990s, however, renders this technique much less valuable than it was in the past.

SAMPLING

Investigators who field community surveys must assure that the individuals who are interviewed in these surveys are representative of the population as a whole. For example, if interviewers were to visit a shopping mall and randomly choose persons in the mall to interview, this would not constitute a representative sample of the population surveyed, even if the mall served an entire community, because people self-select themselves to visit a shopping mall. How does an investigator assure that the sample is as representative as possible? Virtually all community health surveys are household surveys. Yet a household survey, by its very design, immediately creates problems for the investigator wishing to estimate the frequency of psychiatric disorders in a community. Specifically, two groups of individuals in which the frequency of psychiatric disorders is known to be higher would, by design, be missed—the homeless and those residing in long-term care facilities. In addition, household surveys usually do not include college students who are boarding away from home. The Epidemiologic Catchment Area study was a household survey, yet the investigators also included subjects from nursing homes, prisons, and psychiatric hospitals. The homeless, however, were not represented. Thus, a more accurate assessment of psychiatric disorders was possible in the ECA study than would have been possible if a household survey alone had been implemented.

Once a household survey is implemented, how can the investigator be assured that the survey will be representative? The procedures used in the ECA study in North Carolina are instructive. First, the investigators determined that they wished to draw an approximately equal sample of urban and rural subjects. In addition, they wished the sample to be representative of the catchment area in terms of socioeconomic status and racial/ethnic mix. Catchment areas were areas in to which the entire United States was divided during the Community Mental Health Care Movement (CMHC)—i.e., each community Mental Health Center served a specific geographic or catchment area. Census data are available for small, defined areas throughout the United States, and these census data can be used to ensure a representative sample from a catchment area. In the one urban and four rural counties surveyed in North Carolina (two CMHC catchment areas), a number of census-defined areas were selected which ensured that the sample drawn was representative of residency, ethnicity, and socioeconomic status of the five counties.

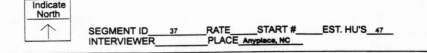

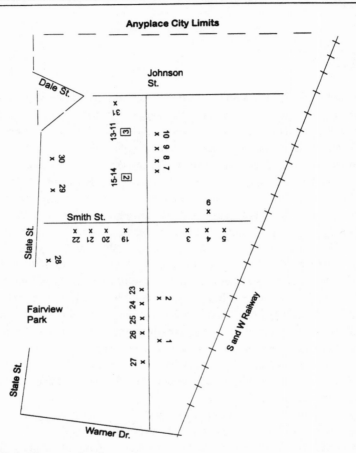

FIGURE 6–1. Segment sketch.

This step in sampling census-defined small areas is referred to as identifying the primary sampling units.

Next, investigators obtained maps for the primary sampling units which contained all streets and known roads (Fig. 6–1). Interviewers then canvassed these primary sampling units and filled in diagrams of every house and other dwelling. Houses were then numbered and a random sample of houses was drawn for each of the enumeration areas throughout the five counties. Investigators assumed that virtually all households would have at least one member 18 years of age or older (the sample was to include persons 18 and older) and that approximately 80% of the persons contacted would participate in the survey. Therefore, for an estimated final sample of 4,000 persons, 5,000 households were selected across the catchment areas, or approximately 20 households across 250 primary sampling units.

In community-based epidemiology studies, an overall response to the survey is usually in the range of 70–80%. Persons not responding to the survey can be categorized as either refusing or never being contacted by the survey interviewers. For example, an interviewer may knock on the door of a house more than once and never find anyone at home.

In a household survey, one approach to selecting sample members is to interview every adult within the house. This approach creates some problems. The sample is not truly "random," for if a household is selected, then all adults in that household are eligible to be interviewed and, if one adult agrees to be interviewed, chances are other adults will agree as well, perhaps at a much higher frequency than if the first adult approached did not agree to participate. In other words, the likelihood of each sample member responding to the survey is not equal across sample members. In addition, the sample is not truly random for it will contain persons related to one another and more persons from homes with multiple adults. For this reason, in most household surveys, such as the ECA, one person is selected from each household.

How does the interviewer know which person to select? Usually a method is employed by which the interviewer has available an algorithm which identifies, in each household, that member of the household who should be interviewed. The interviewer's first task is to determine the age and gender of all adults in the household. For example, if the household contains a married couple, then for one-half of the occasions the husband is selected for the interview and for the other half the wife is selected. Once the sample member is selected, that person is the only individual from that household in the sample. Frequently the person answering the door is not selected as the sample member. The sample member may be away from the household at the time the interviewer determines who lives in the household. The interviewer cannot substitute the person who answers the door (a person who might be quite willing to participate in the survey) but rather must attempt to persuade the person identified by the algorithm to participate.

INTERVIEWING

Selection of interviewers for a community survey is critical to the success of that survey. If the survey does not require clinical expertise, then the best "pool" of persons from which to choose interviewers are persons who have had experience interviewing in the community. At times, inexperienced clinical investigators attempt to perform the interviews themselves. Yet interviews can take 6 to 8 hours to complete and often are performed at night or during the weekend—not a good use of the clinician's time. An excellent pool of interviewers consists of persons who routinely perform census and other community-based interviews. Some investigators have concerns regarding the match of interviewers with subjects, and this is appropriate in certain circumstances. For example, if the survey includes questions regarding sexual abuse, it is frequently appropriate to match the gender of the interviewer with the respondent. In general, the investigator should not worry about matching the interviewers with subjects but rather concentrate upon obtaining the most experienced interviewers possible.

Once interviewers are selected, ample time should be devoted to training them. Training sessions should include both didactic instruction and time for practice with the interview. Interviewers can practice on one another or with actors/actresses who present typical problems interviewers might encounter in the field. Interviewers should be trained to reliability: Two interviewers who interview the same subject and who receive identical information from that subject should record that information identically (see Chapter 10).

For example, the North Carolina ECA investigators selected approximately 50 interviewers to administer the ECA questionnaire, including the DIS. These interviewers were, for the most part, experienced interviewers who had worked in many surveys prior to the ECA. The somewhat complicated structure of the DIS required approximately 40 hours of training by the investigators to ensure reliability before interviewers were assigned households to contact.

Once interviewers are trained, they are assigned a series of households to contact based on the sampling procedures described above. After determining the household composition and using the algorithm described above to identify the subject to be interviewed, the interviewer asks to speak with this individual and encourages the person to participate in the survey. Community-based investigators find that gaining participation of persons in the community has become increasingly difficult because of fears of security among residents of many neighborhoods and the frequent canvassing and surveying, often for promotional purposes, with which they are bombarded. In general, offering special inducements, such as payment, to participate in the interview does not increase participation in surveys. For example, it is often the most wealthy and the most busy who refuse to participate in a survey, and therefore money is little inducement. Rather, appealing to the need to gain information useful to society is the best inducement. If the survey has been publicized, such as through an article in a local newspaper or a television spot, then interviewers can show evidence of the study's credibility. In addition, all interviewers should wear official badges identifying for whom they are working.

Once a subject has agreed to participate, the interviewer attempts to complete the interview in one sitting. Most interviews should be completed in one sitting, and therefore the length of the interview should be no longer than 1 to 2 hours. If for some reason the interview cannot be completed, it is appropriate for the interviewer to return at a later time, but the interval between sessions should be kept to a minimum. Following completion of the interview, the interviewer should check the questionnaire carefully before leaving the home of the subject to make certain that all information was collected appropriately and no questions were missed accidentally. This "first edit" of the questionnaire is followed by a second edit by a research team member other than the interviewer. The second editor carefully reviews the questionnaires before they are forwarded to data entry. Editing a questionnaire is a time-consuming effort. For this reason, many survey investigators now use laptop computers with algorithm-driven questionnaires with response data downloaded onto a disk. Data can be electronically transferred immediately from the disk to the data file, saving hours of labor and making the data available instantaneously for review. Interviewers may give up some flexibility, such as the ability to add marginal notes, with computerized data entry.

The research team must also verify that interviews are actually completed. Therefore a percentage of persons interviewed are called (usually 10–20%) by the study coordinator and asked if they were interviewed and for what length of time the interviewer spoke with the subject. An occasional case of "falsification" of an interview will be discovered. That is, the interviewer may not contact the subject at all or contact the subject only briefly and then fill in the questionnaire as if the subject had answered the questions. When such falsification occurs, all the work of that interviewer becomes suspect.

In the North Carolina ECA study, the interviews were edited by the interviewers following the 1–2 hour interview. At least 3 additional hours were devoted to editing each questionnaire by designated editors before the questionnaire was ready for data entry. In a small percentage of cases (less than 5%), data were missing such that the questionnaire was returned to the interviewer and the interviewer recontacted the subject to ask additional information or to clarify that the subject had initially refused to give the information.

In summary, the process of selecting interviewers, training interviewers, and supervising interviewers during data collection for a community survey is no easy task and is time-consuming. For example, the North Carolina ECA investigators took over 12 months from the time interviewers were selected until the last questionnaires were collected from the interviewers. A "point prevalence" study thus may stretch over many months. This long duration also raises substantive concerns about the validity of the findings. The investigators must assume that there are no seasonal variations in disorders, and no other factors which may significantly change responses to the questionnaire during the survey. For example, if one were performing a mental health survey over a period of time during which a natural disaster occurred in the community surveyed (such as the nuclear accident at Three Mile Island), responses before and after the event might not be comparable.

DATA MANAGEMENT

Before data from a community-based epidemiologic study can be analyzed, the data must be placed in a format which permits analysis. The creation of an accurate and complete data file is central to implementing community-based epidemiologic studies. To ensure accuracy of data entry, data are usually entered twice from the questionnaire, and any discrepancies between the two are compared with the original research instruments to resolve the conflict. Error rates from keying in data are generally in the range of 1–5%, so double entry is essential. If data are entered directly into laptop computers, the software program can eliminate the problems of missing or out-of-range values by refusing to accept certain values or to proceed unless values are appropriate.

A second aspect of data management following data entry is "cleaning the data." Occasionally a value is entered which is inconsistent with other data. For example, gender may be recorded female in one portion of the questionnaire, and responses may suggest a diagnosis of prostate cancer in another portion of the questionnaire. The age of an adult subject may be recorded accidentally as 3. Therefore, investigators apply computer programs to data files in order to identify these problems: The recorded age of "3" would be flagged as an outlier. Most often, these outliers can be resolved by returning to the original questionnaire and perhaps the interviewer. At times, the subject must be recontacted. At other times, however, an outlying value cannot be explained, and the investigator may choose to record this datum as missing. For example, an individual's diastolic blood pressure may be recorded as 400, a value that is so far out of range that it cannot be accepted as accurate, (i.e., a person could not be expected to live with such a diastolic blood pressure). Both these steps in clearing data are eliminated when the data are entered directly into a computer, such as a laptop. Computer-based questionnaires will not accept outliers, and therefore some keying errors are eliminated. Mistakes can still occur, however, as the interviewer enters the data.

Once a clean data set is available, it is put into a format which renders it accessible to analysis. Examples of such data files are Statistical Analysis Systems (SAS) files or Statistical Programs for the Social Sciences (SPSS) files. For large community-based surveys, the amount of data in a file may be so extensive that a desktop computer cannot manage data analysis. This problem is decreasing even as you read, for the capacity of desktop computing continually increases. Even so, in order to render data analysis more feasible, a "work file" is usually created for a particular analysis. These work files extract the variables of interest from the larger file and download them onto a separate computer file for the investigator so that they can be analyzed using a statistical analysis software program such as SAS.

SECONDARY DATA ANALYSIS

Collecting and cleaning data from a large epidemiologic survey is an expensive task. Investigators and funding agencies such as NIMH wish to harvest as much from these data as possible. For this reason, many community-based epidemiologic studies are available for "secondary data analysis" by investigators who were not involved in the initial data collection. Examples of data which are available for public use include the Epidemiologic Catchment Area data (Robins and Regier, 1991) and data from the more recent National Comorbidity Study (Kessler et al., 1994). The entire data set along with a code book can be purchased for a few hundred dollars and set up on a computer locally. An investigator can then engage in secondary analyses. These data sets are excellent resources for young investigators who wish not only to "get their feet wet" analyzing data but also to understand what types of questions can be answered from these large data sets. To ensure that these data sets are used appropriately, the investigator should:

- Obtain a copy of the questionnaire, frequencies of the major variables, and variable names.
- Obtain copies of published articles based on the data set.
- Obtain a thorough description of the methods of the study, including the target population, sampling procedures, and response rates.
- Become familiar with any peculiarities of the study. (For example, the investigators may have oversampled a certain portion of the population.)
- State explicit hypotheses to be tested by the data analysis.
- Lay out proposed tables and figures that are to be generated by the analyses before the analyses are begun.
- Perform preliminary, simple analyses to ensure that the investigator is familiar with the data. For example, previous analyses can be replicated in order to determine if the person performing the secondary analysis obtains the same results as obtained in the original analysis (such as the frequency distribution for a variable).

Secondary analysis is the means by which many young investigators first publish from epidemiologic studies because the number of actual large studies is quite limited. These data sets provide excellent opportunities for young investigators to ask critical questions and analyze data.

DATA ANALYSIS AND PRESENTATION

Most types of analyses reviewed in this book are potentially appropriate to community-based epidemiologic survey data, especially if the survey included follow-up as well as cross-sectional components. Nevertheless, baseline analyses from large community surveys are usually presented in "lead" papers or perhaps in a book describing the survey. For example, though numerous articles have been published from the NIMH ECA Program, an overall description of the program and baseline papers documenting the central findings of the study were published together initially in the October 1984 issue of the *Archives of General Psychiatry*

TABLE 6–1. Prevalence of DIS/*DSM-III* mood disorders by gender and age %(s.e.)

	MEN		WOMEN	
AGE	1 YEAR	LIFETIME	1 YEAR	LIFETIME
18–29	3.1 (.5)	6.4 (.6)	5.8 (.6)	10.6 (.8)
30–44	2.7 (.5)	6.6 (.7)	7.9 (.8)	15.3 (1.0)
45–64	1.7 (.4)	3.6 (.5)	3.6 (.5)	9.3 (.8)
65+	.6 (.3)	1.6 (.5)	1.5 (.4)	3.3 (.6)

From Weissman et al., 1991

(Eaton et al., 1984; Robins et al., 1984; Myers et al., 1984). These findings were later summarized in a book, *Psychiatric Disorders in America* (Robins and Regier, 1991; Weissman et al., 1991). Example of these baseline estimates are presented in Table 6–1. This table is, for the most part, self-evident, but several characteristics should be noted. First, prevalence figures are presented for 1 year and lifetime. One-year prevalence is the prevalence in the year preceding the interview. Lifetime prevalence is the frequency of the disorder that was ever reported by the individual. As would be expected, 1-year prevalence is less than the lifetime prevalence. For a diagnosis of current major depression, a subject may not be depressed at the time of the interview. If he or she recovered from a depressive episode 2 weeks prior to the interview, that subject would be counted as prevalent at both 1 year and lifetime.

The prevalence figures presented in Table 6–1 are "weighted" (see Chapter 12). As noted above, the ECA method assigned each resident in the catchment area a numerical weight which reflected the known probability of that person's being selected for the interview. For example, if only one person in a selected household was 18 years of age or older, that person had a 100% chance of being included in the sample. On the other hand, if four persons 18+ years of age lived in that household, each person in the household had a 25% chance of selection. The North Carolina site oversampled for the elderly: A supplemental group of subjects was selected from the 65+ age group, thus raising the probability of being in the study among elderly persons. It was therefore necessary to adjust the prevalence estimates to account for the varying likelihood of being selected for the sample and, therefore, for the deviations from selecting a simple random sample of the population. These so-called *selection biases* were corrected by weights which were inversely proportional to an individual respondent's relative chance of being selected. Each individual in the sample was assigned a weight, and that weight was used to "weight" the data for all analyses. Weights also adjusted for refusal among certain respondents in relation to age, gender, and race/ethnicity. The use of weights adjusted the analyses such that findings were generalizable to *all* persons 18+ years of age in the five counties surveyed in North Carolina.

Weighting also produces another problem with estimation of prevalence.

Weighted and clustered samples, such as used in the ECA study, have larger overall variances than do simple random samples. If this increased variance is not adjusted downward, the precision of the estimates tends to be exaggerated, and differences may appear statistically significant when in fact they are not. For this reason, standard errors (see Chapter 12) are provided for each prevalence estimate.

Problem Set

A group of investigators visited the homes of 624 students enrolled in a public junior high school in Raleigh, NC, to determine the frequency of major depressive disorder as defined by the Research Diagnostic Criteria (Schoenbech et al., 1982). One hundred twenty students (19%) were not interviewed due to refusal of the parent to give informed consent or refusal of the subject. Data on race/ethnicity of subjects not interviewed were not available. Investigators administered the Center of Epidemiologic Studies Depression Scale (CES-D) to these students (Radloff, 1977). An additional 120 students (19%) did not fill out the CES-D (which was part of a larger questionnaire) or did not answer five or more items from the CES-D.

Eleven (or 2.9%) of the 384 students completing the CES-D reported symptom patterns which, according to investigators, were consistent with RDC major depressive disorder. The investigators concluded from the study that the prevalence of major depressive disorder in students 12 to 15 years of age is similar to that among adults. In addition, the investigators suggest that a self-report questionnaire may be usable to detect a "depressive syndrome" in young adolescents.

Questions

1. What is the population from which this sample is drawn? To what extent do you think this sample is representative? Is the response rate acceptable?

2. Is the use of the self-report symptom scale to approximate a diagnosis of major depressive disorder (using Research Diagnostic Criteria) an appropriate method of case identification?

Answers

1. The population from which this sample is drawn is young adolescents in the urban southern United States. As the sample was limited to a single public junior high school, some may question whether the school would be representative of all schools. The authors' report says that the school is "representative" yet they do not provide evidence for generalizability. Therefore, concern must be expressed regarding the generalizability of this sample.

Three hundred eighty-four responses from a sample of 624 presents problems as well. Therefore a reviewer of this study might have considerable problems accepting this very low response rate (62%). As so little is known regarding depression among young adolescents, however, the study was published in a respected journal.

2. As noted in the chapter text, one use of community surveys is secondary analysis. The original purpose of this survey was not to obtain clinical diagnoses of these adolescents based on RDC criteria. If it had been, the investigators probably would have used an instrument such as the Schedule of Affective Disorders in Schizophrenia (SADS) or the Structured Clinical Interview for DSM (SCID) to make such a diagnosis. Nevertheless, investigators at a later time may attempt to approximate a diagnosis using an instrument not designed to identify cases of a particular diagnosis. The CES-D, given that it is an instrument which asks subjects about symptom frequency during the 1 week prior to the interview(RDC criteria for depression require 1-week duration), provides a potential opportunity to identify cases of major depression. These investigators matched RDC criteria for a depressive syndrome with questions in the CES-D in the appendix of the paper, and the match "looks good,"—i.e., there is face validity to the approach. Face validity exists when the items in a questionnaire "appear" to assess the presence or absence of the symptoms listed in criteria such as the RDC criteria.

The investigators did not validate the use of the CES-D in a separate sample. In other words, the CES-D should have been administered to depressed and nondepressed adolescents previously identified using an instrument such as the SADS. Then the sensitivity and specificity of the instrument in that setting could be presented. Given that these data are not presented, and given that adolescents are not easily diagnosed, one must question the validity of the diagnosis. The authors of this paper recognized the limitation and indicate this in the discussion.

REFERENCES

American Psychiatric Association. 1980. *Diagnostic and Statistical Manual of Mental Disorders, 3rd ed. (DSM-III)*. Washington, DC: American Psychiatric Association.

Bebbington P., Hurry J., Tennant C., Stunt E., Wing J.K. 1981. Epidemiology of mental disorders in Camberwell. *Psychology Medicine* 11: 561–579.

Blazer D.G., Crowel B.A., George L.K. 1987. Alcohol abuse and dependence in the rural South. *Archives of General Psychiatry* 44: 736–747.

Eaton W.E., Holzer C.E., VonKorff M., Anthony J.C, Helzer J.E., George L., Burnam M.A., Boyd J.H., Kessler L.G., Locke B.E. 1984. The design of the epidemiologic catchment area surveys. *Archives of General Psychiatry* 41: 942–948.

Henderson A.S., Duncan-Jones P., Byrne D.G., Scott R., Adcock S. 1979. Psychiatric disorder in Canberra: a standardized study of prevalence. *Acta Psychiatrica Scandinavia* 60: 355–374.

Katz S., Akpom C.A. 1976. A measure of primary sociobiological functions. *International Journal of Health Services* 6: 493–508.

Kessler R.C., McGonagle K.A., Zhao S., Nelson C.B., Hughes M., Esllerman S., Wittchen H., Kendler K.S. 1994. Lifetime and 12-month prevalence of DSM-III-R psychiatric disorders in the United States: results from the National Comorbidity Survey. *Archives of General Psychiatry* 51: 8–15.

Leighton D.C., Harding J.S., Macklin D.B., Macmillan A.M., Leighton A.H. 1963. *The Character of Danger*. New York: Basic Books.

Myers J., Weissman M.M., Tischler G.L., Holzer C.E., Leaf P.J., Orvashel H., Anthony J.C., Boyd J.H., Burk J.D., Cramer M., Stolzman R. 1984. Six-month prevalence of psychiatric disorders in three communities. *Archives of General Psychiatry* 41: 959–970.

Older Americans Resources and Services (OARS). Durham, North Carolina, Duke University Center for the Study of Aging and Human Development, 1978.

The President's Commission on Mental Health: Report to the President from The President's Commission on Mental Health. Washington, DC, stock # 040–000–00390–8, 1978, Vol. 1.

Radloff L.S. 1977. The CES-D scale: a self-report depression scale for research in the general population. *Applied Psychological Measurement* 1: 385–401.

Regier D.A., Myers J.K., Kramer M., Robins L.N., Blazer D.G., Hough R., Eaton W.W., Locke B.Z. 1984. The Epidemiologic Catchment Area program: historical context, major objectives and study population characteristics. *Archives of General Psychiatry* 41: 934–941.

Robins L.N., Helzer J.E., Croughan J., Williams J.B.W., Spitzer R.L. 1981a. NIMH Diagnostic Interview Schedule Version III (May, 1981). Rockville, MD: NIMH MIMO.

Robins L.N., Helzer J.E., Croughan J., Ratcliffe K. 1981b. National Institute of Mental Health Diagnostic Interview Schedule: its history, characteristics, and validity. *Archives of General Psychiatry* 38:381–389.

Robins L.N., Helzer J.E., Weissman M.M., Orvashel H., Grunberg E., Burke J.D., Regier D.A. 1984. Lifetime prevalence of specific psychiatric disorders in three sites. *Archives of General Psychiatry* 41: 949–958.

Robins L.N., Regier D.A. (eds.). 1991. *Psychiatric Disorders in America: The Epidemiologic Catchment Area Study*. New York: Free Press.

Schoenbech V.J., Kaplan B.H., Grimson R.C., Wagner E.H. 1982. Use of a symptom scale to study the prevalence of a depressive syndrome in young adolescents. *American Journal of Epidemiology* 116: 791–800.

Srole L. 1962. *Mental Health in the Metropolis: the Mid-town Manhattan Study*. New York: MacGraw-Hill Book.

Weissman M.M., Bruce M.L., Leaf P.J., Floris L.P., Holzer C. 1991. Affective disorder. In *Psychiatric Disorders in America* (eds. Robins L.H., Regier D.A.), New York: Free Press.

7

LONGITUDINAL STUDIES

OBJECTIVES

- To describe and illustrate longitudinal (or cohort) design in patient-oriented research.
- To distinguish age, period, and cohort effects.
- To describe the strengths and limitations of cohort design.
- To review the most frequently used statistical techniques for longitudinal studies, including relative risk and the life table.

COMMUNITY CASE EXAMPLE

A 16-year longitudinal study of a general population sample in Nova Scotia, the Stirling County Study, began during the early 1950s. One aim of the study was to determine whether the risk of mortality increased in persons experiencing an affective mood disorder. Affective disorder was operationally defined as low spirits accompanied by physical symptoms such as sleep difficulty, loss of appetite, and fatigue and anxiety (a combination of depression disorder and anxiety disorder). Subjects identified as cases of depression had to have experienced these symptoms for at least 1 month and experienced some impairment in work. The baseline prevalence of depression without other syndromes was 1% in men and 2% in women. The frequency of depression with anxiety was 3.7% in men and 4.8% in women.

One thousand three subjects were initially interviewed in 1952 and a baseline diagnosis was assigned by means of a computer algorithm. By mid-1968, 24% of the subjects had died. Subjects who were alive were reinterviewed a second time between 1968 and 1970. The investigators were able to reinterview 618 subjects and make contact with another 57. For the remaining subjects, the investigators searched for death certificates. Then they carried out a third wave of fieldwork to determine the vital status of the subjects for whom they could not find a death certificate. By interviewing and corresponding with relatives, former neighbors, and physicians, and by checking family Bibles and gravestones, the investigators gathered evidence that 242 subjects had died by June of 1968. Of the 227 who died in Nova Scotia, a death certificate was found for all subjects. For the remainder, they were able to obtain a date of death (Murphy et al., 1987). Those with depression were 1.54 times more likely to have died than those without depression.

CLINICAL CASE EXAMPLE

A total of 101 subjects who enrolled in the Psychobiology of Depression Study were followed every 3 months for 1 year after they received a diagnosis of major depressive disorder according to the Research Diagnostic Criteria (RDC). These subjects were not selected randomly, but rather constituted a convenience sample at the several sites participating in the study (Mood Disorders Programs and teaching hospitals such as Harvard, Rush Presbyterian, Washington University, and Pittsburgh). Both inpatients and outpatients were included and many subjects had a long history of mood disorder. Only 50% of the subjects had recovered after 1 year of follow-up. An additional 28% had recovered after two years. In contrast, speed to recovery from entry into the study was more rapid, as 63% of the subjects who recovered during the first year had recovered by 4 months. The recovery rates were about 20% per month for the first 4 months and then declined sharply for the remaining months of the first year of follow-up. Of those who recovered during the first year of follow-up, 24% relapsed within 12 weeks and 12% relapsed within 4 weeks. Factors associated with recovery included superimposition of dysthymia upon the acute episode of major depression, acuteness of onset of the depressive episode, and severity of the episode. Predictors of relapse included an underlying chronic depression and three or more previous affective episodes (Keller et al., 1982a,b).

INTRODUCTION

These two case examples, one from a community population and the other a clinic population, are typical of cohort or longitudinal studies in patient-oriented psychiatric research. The Stirling County Study is one of the best known community-

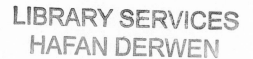

based longitudinal studies in the field of psychiatric epidemiology, and the Psychobiology of Depression Study is the best known longitudinal clinical study of mood disorders in the United States. A cohort study is a study of individuals who are free of disorder (or the outcome of interest) under investigation and who are assigned to groups on the basis of the presence or absence of exposure to a suspected risk factor for the disorder. Participants are then followed over a period of time to assess the occurrence of the disorder or other outcome of interest.

At first glance, the two case examples may not appear to be true "cohort" studies in that a disorder (affective disorders) was present in the cohort when initially surveyed. In the Stirling County Study, however, the outcome of interest was mortality, and individuals initially enrolled in the study had not died. In the Psychobiology of Depression Study, remission and relapse were the outcomes of interest. Both cohorts could also be used to study other outcomes of interest that were not present at baseline. For example, disease-free individuals in the Stirling County Study could be followed for the onset of depression or other psychiatric disorders. Individuals diagnosed with major depression in the Psychobiology of Depression Study could also be followed to determine the factors associated with risk of developing bipolar disorder over time.

There are two types of cohort studies—prospective and retrospective—and both have been applied to psychiatric disorders. In the first type, outcomes of interest have not occurred in subjects at the beginning of the study, and subjects are followed for those outcomes. The most famous prospective study in medicine is the Framingham Heart Study, where all persons enrolled initially were free from cardiovascular disease. Risk factors such as cholesterol levels and hypertension were assessed at baseline to determine which factors contributed to an increased risk for developing cardiovascular disease over many years of follow-up. It was from the Framingham Heart Study that we obtained the first solid evidence that high cholesterol is a risk factor for cardiovascular disease.

In a retrospective cohort study, all outcomes have occurred at the time the study is initiated. Nevertheless, records collected before the outcomes occurred permit the investigator to proceed as if these outcomes were not known. For example, during the early 1970s a group of investigators at the University of Iowa collected mortality data on more than 500 subjects who initially were admitted to the University of Iowa Psychiatric Hospital between 1934 and 1944. They compared these subjects to 160 control patients who had been admitted to a regular hospital for either an appendectomy or a herniorrhaphy. Ninety-seven percent of the subjects had been traced to death or their current addresses by the end of 1974 when the study was completed (Tsuang et al., 1980). The psychiatric patients experienced a higher mortality rate compared to the controls. Both the Framingham and Iowa studies are examples of a cohort design. Further examples of longitudinal or cohort studies in psychiatry are presented in Table 7–1.

THE COHORT DESIGN

This design is illustrated in Figure 7–1 and applied to the Stirling County Study in Figure 7–2. The sample is initially divided into persons with and without the outcome of interest. Persons without the outcome are "at risk" for a disorder, and relative risk is a measure of the probability that a person at risk will become affected during a specified period of time compared to an unexposed person. Then the sample is classified into groups according to their exposure status and followed over time. At follow-up, the presence or absence of disease in the exposed vs. the unexposed category is compared with the total number of persons in the exposed compared to the unexposed categories, thus permitting the calculation of a relative risk of the outcome of interest in the exposed compared to the unexposed group (see Chapter 3). In Figure 7–2, the "disease" is mortality, and therefore all subjects in the sample ($n = 1,003$) were in the "nondisease" category at the beginning of the study. One hundred twenty-one of these subjects were identified as experiencing some type of affective disorder. These individuals were then followed for 16 years and the mortality status of those with affective disorder was compared to that of those with no affective disorder. As shown in Figure 7–2, the relative risk reveals an increased risk of mortality (1.54) for those with a affective disorder compared to those without a mood disorder.

The cohort design has a number of strengths (Table 7–2). It can be quite valuable if the exposure is rare because the sample can be selected on the basis of the exposure status. For example, exposure to lead is thought to contribute to a variety of neurological as well as psychiatric problems. Although exposure to lead is generally rare among children, it is a significant problem among some subpopulations, especially in inner cities. Therefore, a cohort design would be ideal for identifying children at high risk of exposure, such as children living in older housing projects where lead paint was used extensively. The cohort design is also of value in examining multiple effects from a single exposure because multiple outcomes can be assessed over time.

The cohort design is ideal for identifying a temporal relationship between exposure and disease. For example, persons may complain that they experienced major problems with anxiety secondary to emotional trauma, e.g., post-traumatic stress disorder. Identifying the relationship between a stressful event in the past and the onset of anxiety is difficult to establish after the fact. If the trauma can be identified before the onset of symptoms, e.g., the trauma resulting from a railway accident involving hundreds of people, a temporal relationship can be established. Cohort design also permits examination of the effects of changes in exposure status. The best known example in the medical literature is the impact of smoking cessation (compared to continuous smoking) on diseases known to be caused in part by smoking. In the study of psychiatric disorders, persons may be known to

TABLE 7–1. Examples of longitudinal studies

LOCATION: NATION, COUNTY OR CITY	PROJECT DESCRIPTION AND REFERENCE	NUMBER OF SUBJECTS WITH FOLLOW-UP DATA	TOTAL NUMBER OF WAVES	FOLLOW-UP INTERVAL(S) (YEARS)
COMMUNITY STUDIES				
Australia	Prospective study of outcome of depression in elders aged 70+ (Henderson et al., 1997)	936	2	3–4
Canada, Stirling Co., N.S.	Stirling County Study on prevalence and incidence of psychiatric disorders in adults (Murphy et al., 1992)	618	2	16
China, Beijing	Follow-up study of dementia in elders aged 60+ (Li et al., 1991)	825	2	3
Finland, Ahtari	Prospective study of depression in community-dwelling elders aged 60+ (Kivela et al., 1994)	264	2	5
New Zealand	Longitudinal assessment of childhood psychiatric disorders in birth cohort (Fergusson and Lynsky, 1995)	954	16	q. year × 16 years
Sweden, Lundby	Lundby Study on prevalence and incidence of psychiatric disorder in total population (Hagnell, 1989)	2,550	3	10, 25
U.K. (England), Liverpool	Longitudinal study of psychiatric disorder in elders aged 65+, included within Liverpool Studies of Continuing Health in the Community (Copeland et al., 1991)	1,070	ongoing	q. 3 year–death
U.S., Alameda Co., CA	Longitudinal study of depression within Alameda County Study community health study of subjects aged 16–94 (Roberts et al., 1991)	6,928[a]	3	9, 18

Location	Study			
U.S., New York, NY	Midtown Manhattan Panel Study longitudinal study of mental health in urban residents (Srole and Fischer, 1989)	695	2	20

Location	Study			
Colombia, Cali	Follow-up study of adult schizophrenia (Leon, 1989)	101	4	2, 5, 10
India, Agra	Follow-up study of adult schizophrenia (Dube et al., 1984)	62	4	2, 5, 13–14
Nigeria, Ibadan	Retrospective analysis of adult schizophrenia from clinical records (Ohaeri, 1993)	142	2+	7–26
Switzerland, Zurich	Prospective study of all inpatients admitted in one 5-year period with depression, schizoaffective disorder (Angst and Preisig, 1995)	406	6[b]	2, 7, 12,
U.S., Durham, NC	Prospective study of adults aged 29+ with major depressive episode (Blazer et al., 1992)	118	2	1
WHO international study (multiple locations)	World Health Organization Collaborative Study on the Assessment of Depressive Disorders (Thornicroft and Sartorius, 1993)			
Canada, Montreal		100	2	10
Iran, Teheran		57	2	10
Japan, Nagasaki		79	2	10
Japan, Tokyo		81	2	10
Switzerland, Basel		122	2	10

[a]Number of subjects followed up at wave 2; wave 3 follow-up limited to 50% of survivors

[b]Value includes follow-up waves only, because initial admission data for Ss were collected over a 5-year period

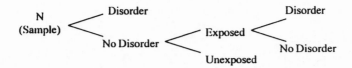

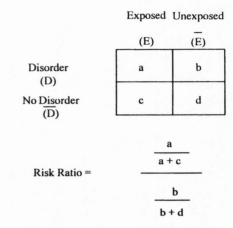

FIGURE 7–1. The cohort design.

have been in a stressful situation, such as the Vietnam War. Some of these individuals may continue in the theater of war for extended periods of time, whereas
others may be deployed for only a short duration. If the persistent (or continual)
exposure to combat leads to adverse mental health outcomes, a comparison of
those who remained exposed over extended periods and those who were removed
from exposure after a brief period provides powerful data to estimate the relationship between exposure and adverse mental health outcome. In addition, the cohort
design minimizes the bias in ascertaining exposure after an event has occurred,
i.e., recall bias.

The cohort design is also ideal when laboratory specimens from a sample have
been stored. Blood samples can be collected at the initiation of a cohort study, and
once markers for psychiatric disorders are identified through molecular biological
explorations, these markers can be assayed in stored blood samples. For example,
Duke University investigators collected blood samples from a cohort of nearly
2,000 older adults in 1992 during a longitudinal study. At about the same time, an
incidence study of dementia was initiated—specifically, Alzheimer's disease.
Since collection of these stored blood samples, a specific allele of apolipoprotein

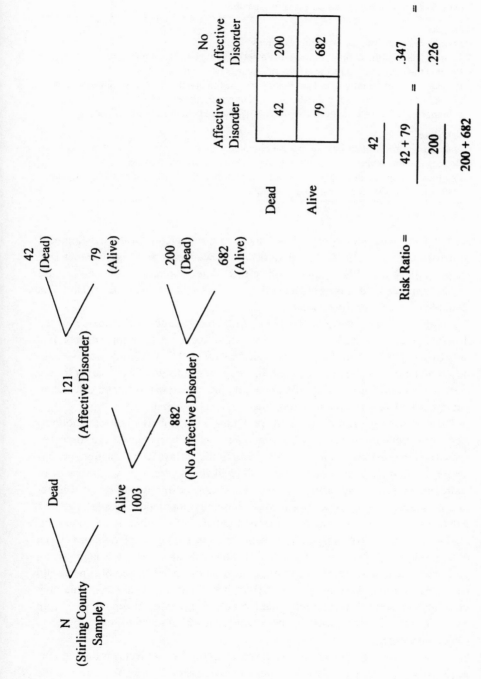

Figure 7–2. The cohort design applied to the Stirling County Study. (From Murphy et al., 1987.)

TABLE 7–2. Strengths and weaknesses of the cohort design

Strengths
- Permits the study of rare exposure variables
- Permits study of the temporal relationship between exposure and disease
- Permits the examination of the effects of changes in exposure status
- Provides the opportunity to collect laboratory specimens, that can be stored until new biological assays relevant to the disease of interest are developed
- Provides data for the direct estimate of risk of disease onset following exposure

Weaknesses
- Not efficient for evaluating rare disease outcomes
- Because many subjects are lost during follow-up, data are incomplete
- Diagnostic methods may change over time, rendering previously collected data incomplete and previous case identification antiquated

E (APOE-4) has been implicated as a significant risk factor for the development of dementia (Roses, 1994). Investigators are now able to genotype samples collected in 1992 for APOE-4 and estimate risk of developing Alzheimer's disease among community-dwelling elders with and without the APOE-4 allele. This is an example of a retrospective cohort design.

Finally, the cohort design permits the direct measurement of incidence of the disease in the exposed and nonexposed and therefore a direct estimate of risk. It is only by using the cohort design that a true "relative risk" of an outcome given exposure to an illness can be calculated. In a case-control study (see Chapter 8), the odds of experiencing a disease if a person reports an exposure can be calculated, but this calculation is only an approximation of relative risk.

The cohort design is not without its problems. First, cohort studies are not efficient for evaluating rare disease outcomes such as rare psychiatric disorders, because over the period of follow-up, few cases of the disease would emerge. For example, in a community-based cohort followed for 1 year, perhaps no cases of anorexia nervosa would emerge. In fact, the cohort design would be an efficient means, when studying a reasonable size community population sample (e.g., $n = 3,000$), to estimate the incidence of only a handful of psychiatric disorders, including the mood disorders, anxiety disorders, and perhaps schizophrenia. Even in a sample of 3,000 persons, the actual incidence of these disorders is relatively rare over 1 year, and therefore follow-up over an extended period of time would be necessary. Given current cost constraints, it is unlikely that samples containing thousands of subjects will be followed for extended periods of time in the future except in rare circumstances. In other words, cohort studies are expensive and time-consuming.

Cohort studies traditionally review a "cross section" of subjects (as did both the Stirling County Study and Psychobiology of Depression Study). Therefore, at the beginning of the study persons have a varied history of psychiatric disorders. For example, in the Psychobiology of Depression Study, some subjects were experiencing their first episode of major depression and others had experienced multiple episodes over many years of enrollment. One approach to eliminating this problem is to enroll persons who are experiencing the first onset of a disorder. In a well-known study sponsored by the World Health Organization, over 1,000 subjects were enrolled at "helping agencies" in 10 countries who were making a first-in-lifetime contact because of symptoms of a psychiatric illness. The outcomes over 2 years were compared and persons from developing countries had a better outcome than persons in developed countries (Sartorius et al., 1986).

Another potential problem with cohort studies is the impact of "lost to follow-up." If investigators cannot maintain contact with persons in the study over extended periods of time, the value of the study is seriously marred because of lost–to–follow-up. In the Stirling County Study, subjects lost to follow-up were rare (a prime reason being that persons did not usually move from Stirling County during their lifetimes). Over 16 years, the investigators learned that of the original 1,003 subjects, 246 had died. For the 97% of the subjects who died in the Canadian Province where Stirling County is located, the investigators were able to locate a death certificate. For the remainder, they were able to determine from an informant the date of death. Sixteen years later, the investigators were also able to reinterview 618 subjects and to make contact with 57 additional subjects who either wished not to participate or who were unavailable for the interview. Therefore, the investigators were able to account for 917 of the original 1,003 subjects, an excellent follow-up over a 16-year time frame.

Yet another problem which plagues cohort studies is especially relevant to psychiatric disorders: Diagnostic methods may change over time. If the definition of a case, e.g., major depression, changes because of changes in the psychiatric nomenclature (the *DSM* manuals), the incident cases will vary in frequency over time depending upon whether the criteria are more or less restrictive. For example, when the Stirling County Study was initiated in 1952, the investigators used a structured interview to assess symptoms of anxiety and depression. A case of severe depression was defined if an individual experienced nervous trouble or a nervous breakdown, low spirits, sleep difficulty, complaints of lowered appetite or tasteless food, fatigue and many ailments, and difficulty with work for at least 1-month duration. These symptoms are somewhat different from the criteria for a major depressive disorder according to *DSM-IV*, in which duration is 2 weeks, and "nervous trouble," poor spirits, and somatic complaints were not included in the diagnostic criteria. Enough similarities exist between old and new psychiatric diagnostic categories so these studies are useful, yet changes in diagnostic criteria significantly influence the generalizability of cohort studies of long duration.

Finally, a potential problem with the cohort design (but also a potential problem with cross-sectional design) is that the sample selected may not be representative of the entire population. The Psychobiology of Depression Study is illustrative.

Subjects entered into this study were "self-selected" in terms of chronicity and severity of their mood disorders. Many of these subjects had experienced previous episodes of severe mood disorders. Therefore one might reasonably question whether the outcome data are generalizable to the typical patient seen for the first time by a psychiatrist and diagnosed with major depression. Perhaps the high propensity to relapse reported would be tempered if a different sample were selected. In other words, a research sample drawn from a specialty clinic in an academic health center may not yield results typical of patients in general psychiatric practices.

SELECTING THE EXPOSED POPULATION

The first step in designing a cohort study is to determine the exposure of interest in the population. Stirling County Study investigators, for instance, were interested in the particular exposure of social disintegration and selected communities in Stirling County that were considered to be socially integrated or disintegrated. In the Psychobiology of Depression Study, the "exposure" was the presence of a diagnosis of major depression. The determination of exposure derives from the research question being asked by the investigators. For example, the Stirling County Study investigators were exploring the relationship between social factors and psychiatric disorders. In the Psychobiology of Depression Study, in contrast, the investigators were interested in the longitudinal course of a major depressive episode.

Selection of the exposed population is also based upon ease of data collection. In the Stirling County Study, individuals lived within a reasonable driving distance of the investigators, and the investigators worked diligently to develop relationships with the community so the study would yield as high a response rate as possible. In the Psychobiology of Depression Study, investigators from those institutions throughout the United States participating in this study enrolled subjects who were attending mood disorder or other outpatient clinics associated with institutions participating in this study. As the Psychobiology of Depression Study was a naturalistic study, i.e., it did not interfere with normal treatment of subjects, this permitted a higher likelihood of follow-up of these subjects than might be expected in a clinical trial (see Chapter 9).

In other cases, the "exposed" population may simply be a population of individuals which is representative of the community at large. The Epidemiologic Catchment Area (ECA) Study (see Chapter 6) is an example of a general population survey in which the sample was reinterviewed 1 year following the initial interview. In this case, depending upon the research hypothesis, a number of subgroups within the population could have been considered "exposed" and compared with persons not exposed. For example, persons divorced during the year prior to the ECA Study but not suffering from a mood disorder could have been compared with nondepressed persons who were married at the time of the survey to determine if a divorce within the year prior to the first interview would lead to an increased risk of a mood disorder during the year of follow-up.

SELECTING THE UNEXPOSED POPULATION

Selection of the comparison group is as important in a longitudinal/cohort study as selection of the exposed population. Most community-based longitudinal studies in psychiatry have begun with a general population or clinic sample and later disaggregated the sample to address specific research questions (such as the ECA studies). In the Stirling County Study, for example, two subgroups within the community sample were selected for comparison, e.g., those who were depressed vs. those who were not depressed. In the Psychobiology of Depression Study, persons with an index episode of major depression were selected as the general cohort for follow-up and then exposure subgroups could be selected. For example, persons with a previous history of depression episodes and others with "double depression" could be compared to individuals with first-onset episodes of major depression.

In other cases, the selection of a comparison group may be more complex. For example, in a community survey of the psychological effects of the nuclear accident at Three Mile Island (an occupational or environmental exposure), the investigators compared the community immediately surrounding the island and a community with very similar characteristics to that of the community near Three Mile Island (in terms of socioeconomic status and work status). They followed these two cohorts over time to determine the incidence of psychological distress (Bromet et al., 1982). At other times, there may be no single comparison group which is similar on all exposure variables except for the variable of interest. In this case, multiple comparison groups may be necessary. For example, if an investigator hypothesizes that a particular neurological disorder is more likely to lead to the onset of major depression than other neurological disorders, that investigator may wish to select multiple comparison groups. The investigator may hypothesize that Parkinson's disease is more likely to lead to major depression than multiple sclerosis, Alzheimer's disease, or a cerebral vascular accident. In such a case, the investigator would choose to compare a cohort of subjects with Parkinson's disease with cohorts of patients experiencing Alzheimer's disease, stroke, and multiple sclerosis.

Some problems arise when a general population sample is used to select a comparison group identified because they have a particular exposure. For example, an investigator may hypothesize that the unemployed are more likely to develop anxiety disorders over time than persons who are employed. Yet the unemployed and employed are different in a number of ways, and therefore a comparison sample of persons mostly employed may not be appropriate. People employed tend to be healthier; they may be differentially exposed to other risk factors for anxiety, such as job stress, and they may seek health care more frequently in case of emergent symptoms because they have health insurance to cover such services, including medications. Therefore, a direct comparison of the general population (most of whom are employed) with those persons not employed may not be a reasonable comparison when considering the likelihood that an individual will develop an anxiety disorder over time.

SOURCES OF EXPOSURE AND OUTCOME DATA

The sources of data for a longitudinal study are somewhat different from a cross-sectional study but less so in most psychiatric epidemiology studies than in general health surveys. Nevertheless, these differences should be indicated. For exposure data, such as a physical illness that predisposes to a psychiatric disorder, medical records may be a useful means for documenting exposure. An investigator, for example, can use medical records to determine if a particular beta blocker is prescribed more often to hypertensive patients who develop major depression than to those who do not develop depression. Interviews and questionnaires are the most frequently used sources of exposure data in psychiatric epidemiologic studies, both cross-sectional and longitudinal, such as were used in the Stirling County Study and the Psychobiology of Depression study.

Physical examinations can be useful sources of data as well: They were used to identify heart murmurs suggestive of mitral valve prolapse in panic disorder. If an investigator proposes that a particular environmental toxin contributes to the onset of a psychiatric disorder, such as lead intoxication leading to mental retardation in children, then direct measures of environmental lead would be the optimal source exposure data.

One means that has been infrequently used to identify an exposure variable (but perhaps will be used more often in the future) is personal monitoring. Suppose that an investigator hypothesizes that inadequate exercise predisposes individuals to develop major depression. Retrospective self-reports of exercise are notoriously inaccurate. Rather, investigators may implement a type of personal monitoring. A motion-sensitive monitor can be placed on the ankle of an individual for a few days, and therefore an estimate of physical activity per day can be accurately obtained for this individual with minimal intrusiveness.

Sources of outcome data also vary in longitudinal studies. As in the Stirling County Study, death certificates usually serve as the most reliable source of mortality status. Medicare records for older persons may be used for determining if individuals have been hospitalized and perhaps institutionalized in long-term care facilities. Hospital records can be used to determine admission to the hospital.

Even so, most psychiatric longitudinal studies use interview data (as used in the Psychobiology of Depression Study) to determine outcome. The follow-up assessments generally can be more brief than the initial assessment and usually are obtained at specified intervals, such as 3 months and 6 months after the initial assessment.

FOLLOWING-UP AND SURVEILLANCE OF COHORTS

In most follow-up studies an important factor is the timing of follow-up, i.e., the follow-up interval. For both the Stirling County Study and the Psychobiology of Depression Study, multiple follow-ups were obtained, and these follow-ups were based on the research questions posed by the investigators. The Stirling County investigators were interested in long-term outcomes such as mortality, and therefore measurement of the final outcome was delayed for many years. In contrast, investigators with the Psychobiology of Depression Study were interested in the longitudinal course of major depression. Given the deterioration in memory for depressive episodes over relatively short periods of time, the investigators selected a 3-month interval for follow-up.

Investigators must constantly weigh the advantages and disadvantages of frequent follow-up. Frequent follow-up provides more accurate information, for the time interval investigated is shorter. Nevertheless, frequent follow-ups are time-consuming, and subjects drop out of studies if follow-ups are so frequent that they become burdensome. Three months, in general, is not too often to recontact subjects enrolled in a longitudinal study. Regardless, these follow-up assessments are difficult, for six or seven attempts to contact a subject may be required before an interview is successfully completed.

Surveillance, in contrast to follow-up of the subject, is the continued monitoring of a population or sample for morbidity and mortality through reported information from health care providers or vital statistics. Surveillance does not require intrusive procedures involving the subject, and interval is based upon the logistics for collecting the data. For example, surveillance for mortality, especially if death certificates are available, can occur at an interval which assures that as many deaths can be accurately documented as possible.

Closely related to fixing an interval of follow-up is the methodology for reducing subjects lost to follow-up. In general, frequent interviews (if these interviews are not perceived as burdensome by the subjects) permit investigators to maintain contact with subjects with such frequent contact that it is unlikely that a subject will leave the area without a trace. Other techniques can decrease loss to follow-up. Birthday cards can be sent to subjects. If the subject has moved, with no forwarding address, the card will be returned to the investigators, who can then use baseline data collected from the subject, such as next of kin and friends, to obtain an updated address. In addition, investigators can use some public records to trace subjects. Using these records, however, may border on invasion of privacy. For example, in most states, motor vehicle records are in theory accessible by investigators, and these records may be used to trace individuals involved in motor vehicle accidents. For mortality data, the National Death Index provides an excellent means for tracing mortality status throughout the United States. In brief, if an investigator knows the social security number, name, date of birth, and last-known residence of an individual, the National Death Index can be scanned each year to determine if that individual has died, even if the individual's current residence is no longer known to the investigator.

Investigators must also keep in mind that there are significant costs to follow-up. Costs accrue when subjects are pursued over significant distances. In studies with relatively few subjects where follow-up of each subject is essential, investigators may budget monies to trace subjects throughout a country or the world. An interviewer may actually fly across country to interview a subject. An example of such a study might be a twin study of Alzheimer's disease where twin pairs, both alive, are identified, one suffering from Alzheimer's disease and the status of the other twin unknown. To determine the status of the cognitive functioning of both twins in order to calculate the hereditary burden of Alzheimer's disease, an in-person interview is essential, regardless of the cost of obtaining the interview. For most community (and clinical) longitudinal studies, however, this type of interview is not feasible. Therefore, investigators must determine over what distance they wish to pursue a subject, that is, the *tracking range*. Investigators may choose to track throughout a state or province, as was done in the Stirling County Study. Cost in future years must also be estimated. Funding for longitudinal studies is not available indefinitely, especially during these difficult economic times. Investigators must plan ahead in terms of their ability to follow subjects over time, even over short periods of time.

BIAS IN COHORT STUDIES

A major source of bias in longitudinal studies is classification bias at the initial evaluation of subjects. For example, in the Psychobiology of Depression Study, if subjects are classified as experiencing a unipolar mood disorder initially, yet they actually suffered from a bipolar disorder, i.e., a previous manic episode had not been identified, then follow-up studies of remission and relapse will be biased. If the initial classification errors are random, then the similarity between two groups will be increased, and a true association would be underestimated. For example, in the Psychobiology of Depression Study, if subjects were equally likely to be misclassified as bipolar when they were in fact unipolar, or classified as unipolar when in fact they were bipolar, this misclassification would decrease the likelihood of identifying a difference in outcome between unipolar and bipolar subjects, such as time from recovery to relapse. Though in this study a misclassification of diagnosis is a misclassification of exposure, diagnostic misclassification is usually a misclassification of outcome. For example, in the Stirling County Study, investigators might have designated incident cases of depression as the outcome and social disintegration as the exposure variable. (In fact, this was the original hypothesis.) Therefore, misclassification of subjects according to whether they lived in socially integrated vs. socially disintegrated communities would be more typical of misclassification of exposure.

Another potential in longitudinal studies derives from nonparticipation at enrollment. Investigators must recognize that those who participate throughout a study are likely to be somewhat different than those who either initially do not agree to enter a study or who become lost to follow-up (or refuse to continue in a study) following the baseline interview. In general, persons who agree to participate and continue to participate are healthier, are more concerned about their health (and in a mental health study, more concerned about their mental health), have better health-related habits, have lower mortality rates, and are more residentially stable. Therefore, the characteristics of initial nonresponders or dropouts (especially mortality status) constitute valuable data because a similarity of characteristics between responders and nonresponders provides confidence that the study findings can be generalized to the entire population. The successful follow-up of the Stirling County participants for mortality status was due to an appreciable effort on the part of the investigators to trace subjects who had moved from the community and dropouts from the study who remained in the community. Otherwise, community residents who continued in the study would have been greatly overrepresented in the sample.

Even though initial response was excellent in this study, the participating subjects were probably somewhat more healthy, both physically and psychiatrically, than persons who refused to participate. Therefore, mortality may have been underrepresented. For these reasons, it is essential to obtain as much information as possible about those individuals who do not participate in a study initially or who are lost to follow-up. In particular, gender, race/ethnicity, and approximate age of initial refusers are often known to investigators and should be examined for difference with participants. A final issue which must be considered in both the design and analysis of a longitudinal study is *confounding*. Confounding can be thought of as the intermixing of the exposure being studied and the outcome with a third factor. The concept of confounding is therefore not limited to the longitudinal design. (It must be taken into account in case-control and clinical trials as well, both at the design and analysis stage.) The importance of understanding confounding, however, can be well illustrated in the longitudinal or cohort design.

In the Stirling County Study, the exposure or independent variable is depression and the outcome is death. A confounding variable is gender, as illustrated in Figure 7–3.

Data from cohort studies yield valuable information about the relative risk (RR)

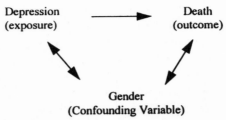

FIGURE 7–3. Interrelationship among exposure, outcome and a confounding variable (gender) in the Stirling County Study. Gender is associated with both depression (depression is more frequent among women) and mortality. (Women have a longer life expectancy.) (From Murphy et al., 1987.)

of developing a disorder in different exposure groups. In their basic structure, the data obtained in a cohort or longitudinal study consists of information about (1) whether or not the individual is exposed to the hypothesized cause of the disorder and (2) the occurrence of the disorder following the exposure (or nonexposure). These data can be simply tabulated in a 2 × 2 table, as illustrated in Figure 7–1. The proportion of all exposed persons who developed the disorder is $a/(a + c)$, and the proportion of all nonexposed persons who developed the disorder is $b/(b + d)$. These proportions or probabilities are compared in the risk ratio (see Chapter 3), a measure of relative risk which is calculated:

$$\text{Risk ratio} = \frac{a/(a + c)}{b/(b + d)}$$

$$= \frac{\text{Cumulative incidence of a disorder in the exposed group}}{\text{cumulative incidence of a disorder in the unexposed group}}$$

When information about person-years of follow-up is also available (see Chapter 3), a different measure of relative risk, the rate ratio, can be used to compare the rate of occurrence among the exposed to the rate of occurrence among the unexposed. It is calculated:

$$\text{Rate ratio} = \frac{a/\text{person-years}}{b/\text{person-years}}$$

$$= \frac{\text{Incidence density of a disorder in the exposed group}}{\text{incidence density of a disorder in the unexposed group}}$$

These measures of relative risk should not be confused with the *odds ratio*, the measure used to estimate risk in a retrospective or case-control study (see Chapter 8). Only in a prospective longitudinal study can true disease rates and individual risk be estimated directly. Relative risk >1.00 indicates an increased vulnerability to an illness given a particular exposure, and a relative risk <1.00 suggests a protective effect. In Figure 7–2, Stirling County Study data are used to calculate the excess risk of mortality for exposed vs. nonexposed subjects: Risk in the affective disorder group was elevated 54% above the risk in the group with no history of affective disorder. If a variable is to confound a relationship, it must be associated with both the independent and/or exposure and the dependent/outcome variable. For example, though female gender is associated with higher frequency of depression, there is no clear evidence that being female causes depression. Female gender may be a surrogate for another factor, such as social stress, which causes depression. In addition, a confounding variable cannot simply be an intermediate link between the exposure and outcome variable—e.g., depression does not lead to increased mortality because depression leads to being female which in turn leads to death.

There are three methods to control for confounding in the design of a study (Hennekens and Buring, 1987). In a clinical trial, confounding can be controlled by randomization (the procedure of choice), which in a large enough study will assure even distribution of the confounding variability across groups. For example, if gender is a potential confounder of response to a medication, then recruitment of enough males and females randomly to the trial will assure even distribution of gender across control and treatment groups. Confounding can also be controlled by restricting certain potential variables. For example, if gender is a potential confounder, restricting a study to females eliminates the potential for confounding even though the study could only be generalized to females. Finally, confounding can be controlled by matching. In matching, the subjects are selected such that the potential confounders (such as age, gender, and race/ethnicity) are distributed identically across groups. A 33-year-old African-American female in the treatment group, for example, could be matched to another African-American female between the ages of 30 and 35 in the control group.

Another approach to analysis in longitudinal studies is the use of the life table, i.e., life-table analysis. The life table summarizes data to describe a pattern of outcome (usually applied to mortality or other discrete events) in populations. The life-table approach was applied to the Psychobiology of Depression Study by Keller et al. (1983) to determine the mean time to recovery from a major depressive episode and subsequently the mean time from recovery to relapse. Proportional hazard models are more sophisticated statistical means to study multiple factors upon the "hazard rate" or the rate at which individuals experience a particular outcome over time. These analyses produce a survival curve.

Longitudinal studies, especially studies that span many years, must be considered from the perspective of age, period, and cohort effects. Age effects are those effects which are known to be age related, such as an increased incidence of Alzheimer's disease in older age groups. Period effects are those events in the sociocultural environment at the time of a study which interact with age and cohort effects and impact an entire population. For example, persons who first sought employment during the economic depression of the 1930s may have been forced to settle for a less desirable job than the sort for which they were qualified. In contrast, those who entered the labor market during the mid-1960s found many jobs available if they were not drafted for the Vietnam War (Atchley, 1985). *Cohort* is a demographic concept which refers to an aggregate of individuals that retains its identity through time, as did the military cohorts in ancient Rome. Cohorts usually are established by year of birth. It is widely known that cohorts born after 1945 have experienced higher suicide rates at all ages compared to cohorts born between 1920 and 1945.

One of the important analytic tasks for the investigator working with longitudinal data over many years is to disentangle age, period, and cohort effects. For example, Schaie (1965) suggests a method to disentangle these influences using multiple analyses from both longitudinal and cross-sectional data, referred to as a *cross-sequential method*. It is not necessary for the purpose of this book to describe the method: What is important is for the reader to recognize that statistical techniques are available to disaggregate these respective influences on psychiatric symptoms and outcomes through time if required data are available (Schaie, 1965).

To take full advantage of sophisticated statistical procedures, such as proportional hazards models, the simple occurrence of an event is not sufficient. Rather, person-years, or person-time, a measurement which sums the cumulative time each person or subject remains in the study before occurrence of the event, is used as the denominator. One advantage of person-years is that subjects who are lost to follow-up in the middle of the follow-up period can contribute data to the analysis for those years during which they were followed.

Problem Set

The "Iowa 500" study is one of the best-known longitudinal studies in psychiatry. The design of the study is unique. During the 1970s, a group of investigators reviewed records from the University of Iowa Psychiatric Hospital between 1934 and 1944. The investigators applied the Feighner Criteria for diagnosis of specific disorders to the well-kept records of symptoms and signs among these hospitalized patients and assigned a research diagnosis to each patient (Feighner et al., 1972). In 1980, Tsuang et al. reported on the results of survival of 200 cases of schizophrenia, 100 of mania, and 225 of depression from the original sample. In addition, they chose from among admissions to the department of surgery at the same medical center between 1938 and 1948 a control sample of 160 hospitalized surgical patients who had an appendectomy or herniorrhaphy who had no psychiatric symptoms. The control group was matched to the psychiatric cases for age at admission, gender, and admission pay status (public or private). By the end of 1974, the investigators had traced 97% of the study subjects (663 out of 685) to death or their current address. Of the study subjects, 54% were dead and 43% were living (3% not traced). Tsuang and colleagues found excess early mortality among the schizophrenics, manics, and depressed patients compared with the surgical patients. Factors associated with shortened survival included diagnostic group, gender, age at admission, and pay status at admission. The excess causes of death were suicides, accidents, and infection and circulatory system diseases. Life-table and proportional hazards analysis were used in this study, controlling for age and gender.

Questions

1. What design was used in this study?
2. Why do you believe the investigators were so successful in tracing the status of subjects in the study after 30 to 40 years?
3. Can you draw a rough approximation of what you believe a survival curve would look like for this study?
4. Are there problems in generalizing from this sample?

Answers

1. These investigators used a retrospective–prospective design. All of the data needed for the study were available at the time the investigators began the study. The diagnoses (exposure status) were derived from data prior to any deaths and applied to subjects independent of knowledge of ultimate mortality status.
2. The investigators took advantage of the stability of the population in Iowa. Very few persons moved out of the state, and the state kept accurate records of death. It would be almost impossible to perform this study in New York City given the mobility of the population.
3. A survival curve is presented in Figure 7–4. Along the horizontal axis, one usually plots the time from the onset of the study in years or months, as was the most appropriate unit in the Psychobiology of Depression Study where the time

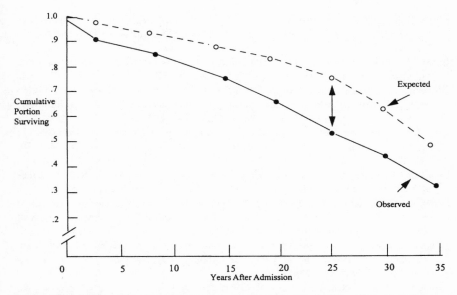

FIGURE 7–4. Observed and expected survival curves for female ($N = 123$, right) depressives. Double-headed arrows indicate maximum differences in curves (females, .184; significant at $p \le .05$). Critical value was .110 for females (From Tsuang et al., 1980.)

interval to the event of interest was greatly shortened. Along the vertical axis the cumulative proportion of the subjects surviving is plotted. Using sophisticated statistical techniques, the investigators can calculate the expected survival curve and then compare that with the observed survival curve to determine if the curves are significantly different from one another.

4. Yes. The results cannot be generalized to all schizophrenics, manics, and depressives. For example, the likelihood of being hospitalized for a psychiatric disorder in Iowa may differ from the likelihood from being hospitalized for a similar disorder in another state, perhaps due to availability of outpatient care. In addition, since the Iowa sample was almost entirely Caucasian, it is not certain that results can be generalized to other race/ethnic groups. Yet the Iowa psychiatric facility was one of the few psychiatric facilities in the state at that time and admitted both public and private patients, and this renders the results more generalizable than would be the case for a typical public, state-supported facility of the sort prevalent during the 1930s.

REFERENCES

Angst J., Preisig M. 1995. Course of a clinical cohort of unipolar, bipolar and schizoaffective patients: results of a prospective study from 1959 to 1985. *Schweizer Archiv fur Neurologie und Psychiatrie* 146: 5–16.

Atchley R.C. 1985. *Social Forces in Aging: An Introduction to Social Gerontology*, p 12. Belmont, CA: Wadsworth.

Blazer D.G., Hughes D.C., George L.K. 1992. Age and impaired subjective support: predictors of depressive symptoms at one-year follow-up. *Journal of Nervous and Mental Disease* 180: 172–178.

Bromet E., Schulberg H.C., Dunn L. 1982. Reactions of psychiatric patients to the Three Mile Island nuclear accident. *Archives of General Psychiatry* 39: 725–730.

Copeland J.R., Dewey M.E., Saunders P. 1991. The epidemiology of dementia: GMS-AGECAT studies of prevalence and incidence, including studies in progress. *European Archives of Psychiatry and Clinical Neuroscience* 240: 212–217.

Dube K.C., Kumar N., Dube S. 1984. Long term course and outcome of the Agra cases in the National Pilot Study of Schizophrenia. *Acta Psychiatrica Scandinavica* 70: 170–179.

Feighner J.P., Robins S.E., Guze S.B., Woodruff R.A., Winokur G., Munoz R. 1972. Diagnostic criteria in psychiatric research. *Archives of General Psychiatry* 26: 57–63.

Fergusson D.M., Lynsky M.T. 1995. Childhood circumstances, adolescent adjustment, and suicide attempts in a New Zealand birth cohort. *Journal of the American Academy of Child and Adolescent Psychiatry* 34: 612–622.

Hagnell O. 1989. Repeated incidence and prevalence studies of mental disorders in a total population followed during 25 years: the Lundby Study, Sweden. *Acta Psychiatrica Scandinavica* 79 (*Suppl.* 348): 61–77.

Henderson A.S., Korten A.E., Jacob P.A., Mackinnon A.J., Jorm A.F., Christensen H., Rodgers B. 1997. The course of depression in the elderly: a longitudinal community-based study in Australia. *Psychological Medicine* 27: 119–129.

Hennekens C.H., Buring J.E. 1987. *Epidemiology in Medicine*. Boston: Little Brown, 1987.

Keller M.B., Shapiro R.W., Lavori P.W., Wolfe N. 1982a. Recovery and major depressive disorder: analysis with the life table and regression models. *Archives of General Psychiatry* 39: 905–915.

Keller M.B., Shapiro R.W., Lavori P.W., Wolfe N. 1982b. Relapse and major depressive disorder: analysis with the life table. *Archives of General Psychiatry* 39: 911–915.

Kivela S.-L., Kongas-Saviaro P., Kesti E., Pahkala K., Laippala P. 1994. Five-year prognosis for depression in old age. *International Psychogeriatrics* 6: 69–78.

Leon C.A. 1989. Clinical course and outcome of schizophrenia in Cali, Colombia: a 10-year follow-up study. *Journal of Nervous and Mental Disease* 177: 593–606.

Li G., Shen Y.C., Chen C.H., Zhau Y.W., Li S. R., Lu M. 1991. A three-year follow-up study of age-related dementia in an urban area of Beijing. *Acta Psychiatrica Scandinavica* 83: 99–104.

Murphy J.M., Monson R.R., Olivier D.C., Sobol A.M., Leighton A.H. 1987. Affective disorders and mortality: a general population study. *Archives of General Psychiatry* 44: 473–480.

Murphy J.M., Monson R.R., Olivier D.C., Zahner G.E., Sobol A.M., Leighton A.H. 1992. Relations over time between psychiatric and somatic disorders: the Stirling County Study. *American Journal of Epidemiology* 136: 95–105.

Ohaeri J.U. 1993. Long-term outcome of treated schizophrenia in a Nigerian cohort: retrospective analysis of 7-year follow-ups. *Journal of Nervous and Mental Disease* 181: 514–516.

Roberts R.E., Lee E.S., Roberts C.R. 1991. Changes in prevalence of depressive symptoms in Alameda County: age, period, and cohort trends. *Journal of Aging and Health* 3: 66–86.

Roses A.D. 1994. Apolipo protein E affects the rate of Alzheimer's disease expression: beta-amyloid burden is a secondary consequence dependent on APOE genotype in duration of disease. *Journal of Neuropathology and Experimental Neurology* 53: 429–437.

Sartorius H., Jablensky A., Korten A., Ernberg G., Anker M., Cooper J.E., Day R. 1986. Early manifestations and first-contact incidence of schizophrenia in different cultures. A preliminary report on the critical evaluation phase of the WHO Collaborative Study on determinants and outcomes of severe mental disorders. *Psychological Medicine* 16: 909–928.

Schaie K.W. 1965. A general model for the study of developmental problems. *Psychological Bulletin* 64: 92–107.

Srole L., Fischer A.K. 1989. Changing lives and well-being: the Midtown Manhattan panel study, 1954–1976. *Acta Psychiatrica Scandinavica* 79 (Suppl. 348): 35–44.

Thornicroft G., Sartorius N. 1993. The course and outcome of depression in different cultures: 10-year follow-up of the WHO Collaborative Study on the Assessment of Depressive Disorders. *Psychological Medicine* 23: 1023–1032.

Tsuang M.T., Wolson R.F., Fleming J.A. 1980. Premature deaths in schizophrenia and affective disorders: an analysis of survival curves affecting the shortening survival. *Archives of General Psychiatry* 37: 979–983.

8

CASE-CONTROL STUDIES

OBJECTIVES

- To describe the design of a case-control study and its advantages and disadvantages.
- To describe common strategies for selecting psychiatric cases and sources of misclassification of psychiatric cases.
- To describe common strategies for assembling optimal noncase (control) groups.
- To identify sources and dimensions of data on exposures and the advantages and disadvantages of different approaches to quantifying exposure data.
- To estimate the relative odds of an exposure among psychiatric cases as compared to noncases.
- To identify the appropriate modeling procedures for controlling confounding factors when estimating the odds of an exposure among cases and noncases.

CASE EXAMPLE

Approximately 15% of all patients treated with neuroleptic agents manifest some form of tardive dyskinesia (TD), but the prevalence of severe cases (characterized by incapacitating involuntary movements) is relatively low. For this reason, and because it is relatively difficult to categorize patients by level of symptom severity, studies of severe TD are scarce. Yassa et al. (1990), in order to "identify treatment variables associated with severity of tardive dyskinesia" (p. 1156) compared case groups of patients with different levels of symptom severity. Initially, they enrolled a large sample ($n =$ 558) of inpatients and outpatients who had used neuroleptic agents for at least 2 years. The Simpson Rating Scale (SRS) (Simpson et al., 1979) was used to determine whether subjects met criteria for TD, and to rate the symptoms of all subjects with TD as severe, moderate, or mild. Because the investigators were examining the correlates of TD severity (as opposed to the presence or absence of TD), they selected for further analysis only subjects meeting criteria for TD for whom complete medical records were available ($n = 155$). In some analyses, patients with severe or moderate TD were grouped together (cases) and compared to patients with mild TD (controls). Yassa et al. then determined the frequencies of various exposure factors (including presence of comorbid organic disorders and treatment history variables) for each of these two groups. In these analyses, prevalence of most health-related factors (e.g., cardiovascular disease, diabetes, insulin coma) did not differ between cases and controls, but the odds of mental retardation were significantly higher in the case group.

THE CASE-CONTROL DESIGN

In a case-control study, individuals who have a disorder or a symptom profile such as severe tardive dyskinesia are identified as *cases*. They are then compared to individuals who do not have the disorder (*controls*) with respect to their history of exposure to a risk factor. The case-control study is a strategy for inferring the cause of a disorder by first identifying its putative effect. Thus, subjects are first identified as affected or not affected by the disorder (cases or controls) and then identified as exposed or not exposed to the risk factor. Case-control studies differ from cohort studies by virtue of this categorization into at least two groups of subjects, cases and noncases, followed by the assessment of exposure level in the two groups. In contrast, as shown in Figure 8–1, cohort studies categorize subjects from a single population as exposed or not exposed and follow both groups forward in time, either retrospectively or prospectively, to the determination of case or noncase status.

Why would an investigator choose to explore a cause-and-effect relationship using a case-control design? When one is studying psychiatric disorders of low prevalence, the primary benefit of a case-control study is efficiency with respect to time and resources. A case-control design allows investigators to identify and assemble the available cases of a disease along with a similar group of persons who have not manifested the disease and to compare them with respect to past exposure to a putative cause or causes.

In the example, Yassa and colleagues were able to assemble a sizable group of

CASE-CONTROL STUDY

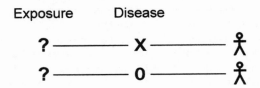

RETROSPECTIVE COHORT STUDY

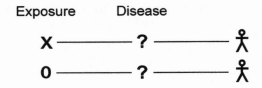

PROSPECTIVE COHORT STUDY

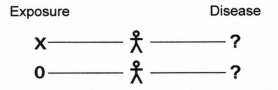

FIGURE 8–1. Comparison of study designs: case-control study, retrospective cohort study, and prospective cohort study.

severe TD patients for comparison to moderately and mildly affected patients. A less efficient strategy would have been to follow large numbers of patients treated with neuroleptics prospectively over time until one had accrued enough severe cases to draw valid conclusions about correlates of severe disease. Table 8–1 lists other advantages and disadvantages of case-control studies which are discussed in this chapter.

TABLE 8–1. Advantages and disadvantages of a case-control design

Advantages
• Faster than longitudinal or cohort study
• Less expensive due to smaller sample size
• Suitable for study of rare diseases
• Suitable for study of a range of independent or interacting exposures
• Confidence intervals acceptably small

Disadvantages
• Less suitable for study of rare exposures, unless rare exposure causes a high proportion of cases
• Less suitable for study of diseases for which medical care is not sought
• Cannot compute absolute exposure-specific rates or risks, only the ratio of rates or risk in two groups (cf. Chapter 3)
• Highly susceptible to bias

DEFINING A CASE

Because the case group should include only true cases, preventing misclassification of cases is a high priority. If a case group includes false cases, the relationship between the exposure and disorder in question will be underestimated.

Mixing true and false cases in psychiatric case groups occurs for several reasons. Psychiatric disorders are based on clinical signs and symptoms that represent heterogeneous underlying pathophysiological and psychosocial causes. Sometimes, therefore, there is no consensus on the criteria for "caseness," and a subject may be considered a case according to one set of criteria but not according to another. Yassa et al. (1990) used the Simpson Rating Scale, but other investigators consider the Abnormal Involuntary Movements Scale or AIMS (US-NIMH, 1975) to be the standard for identifying cases of TD. Furthermore, within any one scale, determination of "caseness" can be problematic when signs and symptoms are reported differently by the subject (case), family members, psychiatrists, or other health professionals. For example, two psychiatrists may rate the same patient differently when using the AIMS.

Mixing true and false cases also occurs when the disorder has a continuum of severity, such as tardive dyskinesia or generalized anxiety. If mild cases are included, a large case group is easier to assemble, but the chance is greater of inadvertently mixing noncases with cases since diagnosis in the early stages of many disorders is imprecise. If only severe cases are studied, the case group may not represent persons who never progressed beyond a mild expression of the disorder or persons who had severe cases of the disorder but died before enrollment.

Yassa and colleagues (1990) briefly discussed three possible ways to identify TD cases: a subjective patient rating of distress or functional impairment, the Simpson

Rating Scale (SRS) for individual body areas, and a cumulative SRS severity score. The SRS scale depends on a trained observer who reports the presence and severity of 34 types of movements in seven body areas using a scale of 1 (no tardive dyskinesia) to 6 (severe tardive dyskinesia). Neither the contents, nor the scaling, nor the validity, nor the reliability of the SRS was discussed, even though the SRS is much less widely known among psychiatrists than the Abnormal Involuntary Movement Scale (AIMS) for assessing the severity of tardive dyskinesia.

Heterogeneity of the case group can arise if cases are drawn from all patients affected at a specific moment in time (e.g., prevalent cases in a cross-sectional study) instead of enrolling cases as they are newly diagnosed (incident cases). Prevalent case groups are less desirable, as they are likely to display mixed effects of exposures related to the onset of a disorder (risk factors) with exposures related to its course (prognostic factors). For example, a first episode of major depression, untreated at time of diagnosis, is much different than a 10th episode which breaks through prophylactic pharmacotherapy and may have different precipitating factors. Incident cases are also preferable if past exposures are to be self-reported, because there is minimal time for knowledge of the diagnosis to have created an enhanced memory of the exposure or an alteration in exposure level, either of which would introduce differences between cases and controls in ways which are not truly related to the antecedent causes of the disease.

Several other strategies are appropriate to determining caseness. To the extent that a causal pathway may be hypothesized, case groups should be defined with an eye toward a homogeneous etiologic entity and not toward a broadly representative clinical sample. Yassa and colleagues were particularly interested in characterizing correlates of severe TD, in distinction to mild or moderate TD, which was more prevalent in clinical samples, and therefore strictly limited their case group to those severely affected. Multiple case groups representing different criteria or different sources of information or different severity levels can also be compared to control subjects for the most nuanced comparisons of risk in different case groups.

OPERATIONALIZING THE CASE DEFINITION

Once a case has been defined conceptually, the investigator must define the case group in practical terms. How can an investigator assemble a group of cases? Because no study can enroll all cases, the investigator begins by identifying an available subpopulation of cases, such as all patients with a diagnosis of TD who attend a mental health clinic or all residents of nursing homes in a specific city who have a diagnosis of TD. These constitute the sampling frame, from which a systematic random sample of units is drawn. Even a random sampling of available subjects will not ensure an unbiased estimate of effect if the total group of available subjects differs from the entire population of cases to which one wishes to generalize, due to some constraint of time, geography, or use of medical care. Generalizability can also be problematic if the case group is too heterogeneous. For example, if an investigator wishes to study the risk factors for vascular depression, the case group should be purged of depressed patients with measurable cognitive impairment, a condition which may share risk factors with vascular depression while being etiologically distinct. Common strategies for selecting cases are outlined in Table 8–2.

The advantages and disadvantages of various sources for cases are presented in Table 8–3. Cases drawn from nursing homes may have more comorbid conditions, be in a later stage of the disease, or have more generous insurance coverage than noninstitutionalized cases. Cases drawn from medical records also may be nonrepresentative when the disease is stigmatized. Case groups drawn from the community, such as community mental health center patients, may present their own set of limitations, particularly when refusal rates are usually high in noninstitutionalized samples of persons with psychiatric problems.

In the case example of severe TD, study participants were chronic ward inpatients or outpatients of Douglas Hospital, Montreal, who had used neuroleptic agents for 2 years or more, and whose diagnoses of schizophrenia were made according to *DSM-III*. The type of hospital is not stated and may be a general service or psychiatric institution or a community-based or a referral hospital. The investigators did not inform the reader whether the total population of eligible patients was enrolled or only a subsample, what the primary or comorbid diagnoses of the subjects were, or the extent to which all affected citizens of Montreal were equally likely to be treated or referred for psychiatric illness.

The authors decided that both the subjective patient rating scale and the cumulative SRS score were too restrictive, reasoning that (1) patients seldom complain

TABLE 8–2. Common strategies when selecting cases

- Define the sampling frame using:
  - Death certificates
  - Population registries
  - Inpatient, outpatient, or long-term care medical records
  - Pathology logs
  - Single or multiple sites or facilities
  - First admission (incident cases) or subsequent admission (prevalent cases)

- Use all cases from a population, if possible. Alternatively, draw a random sample of all cases from a population

- Develop clear and reproducible selection criteria, including inclusion and exclusion criteria
  - Report frequencies for eligibility and loss to follow-up
  - Use multiple case groups where criteria are uncertain

- Aim for a homogeneous etiologic, rather than a representative, case group

---

TABLE 8–3. Advantages and disadvantages of particular case groups

Cases obtained from medical records
  Advantages
  • May be the most accessible group of affected persons
  Disadvantages
  • May be nonrepresentative of all affected persons
  • May be difficult to characterize nonrepresentativeness
  • May miss nonusers of medical care if disease is not serious
  • May overselect patients in late stage of disease if hospital is a referral center

Cases obtained from community surveys
  Advantages
  • May be most representative of total population of affected persons
  Disadvantages
  • May be susceptible to misclassification if diagnostic criteria depend on treatment
  • May be susceptible to refusals, making interpretation of findings difficult

Prevalent cases (vs. incident cases)
  Advantages
  • May provide the greatest number of cases in the least amount of time
  Disadvantages
  • May include differential disease stages
  • May permit altered exposure levels postdiagnosis
  • May confuse factors related to onset with factors related to course

about their movements and (2) subjects with very severe TD in one body area might have low total body scores. Instead, cases were operationally defined as eligible subjects who received a SRS score of 5 (moderately severe) or 6 (severe) in at least one body area.

Cases are sometimes identified from among subjects in a preexisting cross-sectional (Chapter 6) or cohort (Chapter 7) study. This design is called a *nested case-control study.* The advantage of identifying cases (and controls) nested within a cohort design is that in such a study exposures are measured prior to the detection and diagnosis of a disorder. Thus the extent of the exposure may be more accurately assessed and recorded than would be in the case of past exposures for which the respondent would be required to remember back over some considerable time frame. The advantage of identifying cases (and controls) nested within a cross-sectional design is reduced expense associated with identifying controls.

DEFINING CONTROLS

Selecting controls is one of the most difficult tasks in a case-control study. The control group contains persons at risk of developing the disorder who had not become affected at the time of their selection. In the case example, Yassa et al. treated subjects with mild TD as controls. These controls had been treated with neuroleptics and were therefore considered to be at risk for moderate or severe TD.

The control group or groups are compared to the case group with respect to the exposure of interest. All other factors being identical, both cases and controls would be expected to report the same prevalence of the exposure if there were no association between the exposure and disorder. Thus, for example, schizophrenic patients with moderate-to-severe TD would be expected to report similar histories of ECT treatment if there were no relationship between ECT treatment parameters and severity of TD. Common strategies and problems related to the selection of controls are listed in Table 8–4.

Control subjects should be as similar as possible to cases with the exception of their exposure level to the primary risk factor of interest. Control subjects are often unaffected patients in the same hospital or clinic, unaffected friends or neighbors referred by the case group, or unaffected members of the same community from which a case has been identified (Table 8–5). Hospital controls, the most convenient comparison group for hospital cases, are generally assumed to share similar referral patterns and quality of exposure data, although this is rarely tested empirically. For example, if cases are hospitalized schizophrenics, then hospitalized patients with social phobia might not represent an optimum control group because their likelihood of hospitalization is much lower and their memory for past exposure is much better than that of schizophrenics.

TABLE 8–4. Common strategies when selecting controls

- Aim for an estimate of the exposure rate expected to occur in cases if there were no association between the study disorder and exposure. In the absence of an etiological relationship between exposure and disorder, the control group should report the same prevalence of the exposure as the case group

- Use equivalent selection criteria, including inclusion and exclusion criteria, for controls and cases

- Define clearly the sample frame using either a probability sample of unaffected individuals from the same community, enumerated with:
  - Random digit dialing
  - Population registries
  - Voting lists
  - Door-to-door canvassing
  or patients at the same institutions as cases with conditions of comparable severity but believed to be unrelated to the exposure (e.g., incident disorders from the same psychiatric service but unrelated to exposure)

- Exclude a control:
  - With a similar disorder which is potentially related to the exposure of interest
  - With a similar disorder if that disorder could have caused controls to alter their exposure level

TABLE 8–5. Advantages and disadvantages of particular control groups

Controls obtained from community surveys
Disadvantages
• May be less motivated to participate
• May be more expensive and difficult to enroll or assess

Institutional controls
Advantages
• May be easily identified in sufficient numbers
• May have similar awareness of risk factors as cases
• May be similarly willing to cooperate as cases
• May present similar acuity level as cases
• May equalize impact of hospitalization on interview
• May balance selection bias
Disadvantages
• May differ from healthy controls on factors related to exposure
• May differ from source population of cases
• Risk factors may overlap between disorders

Neighbors or co-workers of the cases
Advantages
• May approximate geographical mix of cases
Disadvantages
• May differ in use of health care services, such as use of a different hospital or clinic
• May be less motivated to participate
• May have similar risk factors as cases

   In the case example of severe TD, controls were identified based on the administration of the SRS by the first author to all eligible subjects. Having a single rater with a single scale in a single hospital determine control vs. case status minimizes any potential differences in categorizing cases and controls associated with multiple raters or multiple scales. However, the investigators did not discuss the training of the single rater in the use of the rating scale or state whether that rater, although a practicing psychiatrist in that hospital, was completely blinded to exposure status when rating patients on severity of TD.
   Use of friends or neighbors of cases is a quick and easy way to accumulate controls, but refusal rates may be higher than among hospital controls, and cases may refer friends not randomly but based on some factor associated with the exposure of interest. Community controls may be sampled from tax or voting lists or by telephone random-digit dialing, but the appropriateness of this method may be problematic if the research questions posed are related to demographic, socioeconomic, or health behavior factors which are—in turn—reflected in property ownership, voting behavior, or telephone subscription. Examples of the variety of control groups used by investigators of psychiatric illness are presented in Table 8–6.

TABLE 8–6. Examples of control subjects in psychiatric investigations

EXPOSURE / HYPOTHESIS	CASES	CONTROLS	MATCH
Reduced cerebral glucose metabolism distinguishes attention-deficit hyperactivity disorder (ADHD) (Zametkin et al., 1993)	Adolescents with ADHD ($n = 10$)	Normal adolescents without ADHD ($n = 10$)	Sex, age
Family history of psychosis distinguishes early onset affective disorder (Guth et al., 1993)	Adults with affective disorder and a history of childhood depression ($n = 47$)	Adults with affective disorder and no history of childhood depression ($n = 47$)	Sex, class, ethnicity
Impaired cell-mediated immunity distinguishes subtypes of major depressive disorder (MDD) (Hickie et al., 1993)	Adults with MDD and melancholia ($n = 31$); adults with MDD and no melancholia ($n = 26$)	Normal adults ($n = 31$) Normal adults ($n = 26$)	Both sets of controls matched for age, sex
Risk of schizophrenia is higher among Afro-Caribbean persons (Wessely et al., 1991)	First-contact schizophrenic patients ($n = 130$)	First episode nonpsychotic psychiatric patients ($n = 130$)	Age, sex, period
Sexual abuse increases risk of bulimia nervosa in women, is specific to bulimia nervosa, and varies by referral status (Welch and Fairburn, 1994)	Community-based subjects (Ss) with bulimia nervosa ($n = 50$)	Community Ss w/o eating disorder ($n = 100$); community Ss w/o eating disorder but w/ other psychiatric disorder ($n = 50$); secondary clinical referrals for bulimia nervosa ($n = 50$)	Age (all control groups), social class of parents (for community-based control groups only)

(continued)

TABLE 8–6. (*Continued*)

EXPOSURE / HYPOTHESIS	CASES	CONTROLS	MATCH
Negative life events, heredity, and social support are associated with Graves' disease (Winsa et al., 1991)	Adults with incident Graves' disease in a population of 1,000,000 (n = 208)	Unaffected adults (n = 372) selected from same population register; initially 2 matched controls per case	Sex, age, current county of residence
Specific mental disorders and co-morbidity distinguish young male suicides (Lesage et al., 1994)	Young men aged 18–35 whose deaths were confirmed suicides (n = 75) (data from key respondents, medical records)	Living young men (n = 75) (data from key respondents, medical records)	Age, occupation, marital status, neighborhood
Rapid cycling modifies the course of bipolar disorder (Bauer et al., 1994)	Adults with bipolar disorder and 4+ episodes/ 12 months (n = 120), pooled from 4 sites	Adults with bipolar disorder and 0–3 episodes/ 12 months (n = 119), pooled from 4 sites	—
What demographic and clinical factors increase the risk of visual hallucinations among macular degeneration patients? (Holroyd et al., 1992)	All patients reporting visual hallu-cinations (n = 13) from a series of 100 consecutive Ss with age-related macular degeneration	For each case, the next 3 macular degeneration patients without visual hallucinations from the same series were selected as controls	—

RATIO OF CASES TO CONTROLS

When choosing controls, the question arises: How many controls are needed? Control subjects are often expensive to identify, enroll, and assess, so investigators need only enough controls to ensure statistical efficiency and the probability that a representative range of exposures will be observed (Table 8–7). When the number of available cases is limited, increasing the number of control subjects (relative to cases) up to 4:1 can improve the statistical power of the study (Gail et al., 1976) (see Chapter 9). If some of the available controls may actually have the disorder (i.e., be misclassified as controls) because they did not necessarily seek treatment in the facility from which cases were identified, increasing the number of controls dilutes the effect of misclassification.

If an investigator believes that one source of control subjects may introduce certain kinds of bias into the study, then using two or more control groups is warranted. If several control groups are used and if the estimates of effect are similar across multiple comparison groups, the validity of inferences made about the whole population of exposed persons is enhanced.

Matching (pairing one or more controls to each case with respect to specified characteristics such as age and gender) has been used as a strategy to minimize some of the differences between cases and controls, but matching procedures may introduce more problems than they solve (Rothman, 1986).

In the case example, Yassa and colleagues rated 191 (34%) of 558 psychiatric patients as positive for tardive dyskinesia in one or more body areas. Of these, 20 exhibited severe TD, 80 exhibited moderate TD, and 91 exhibited mild TD, for a total $n = 191$. Of these 191, 36 (19%) had incomplete charts and were omitted from the analyses. Omitted patients did not differ from included subjects on age, gender, primary diagnosis, or age of first exposure to neuroleptics. Among the 155 (81%) with complete medical records, there were 19 severe cases, 70 moderate cases, and 66 with mild TD. In some analyses, the authors elected to combine severe and moderate cases into a single case group and compared them to mild cases as the control group. Participation rates for the initial and study samples are displayed in Figure 8–2.

TABLE 8–7. Ratio of cases to controls

- Use 1:1 controls-to-cases
  When controls are highly available and cost of recruitment is similar for cases and controls

- Use up to 4:1 controls-to-cases
  When cases are limited and expensive to recruit and test
  When controls may be misclassified because they were not seen in a treatment facility

- Use multiple control groups when possible
  To compare differences in magnitude of associations and/or rule out effect of bias

---

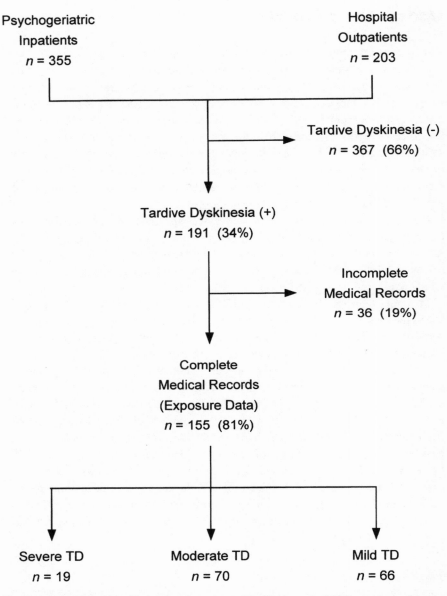

FIGURE 8–2. Flow chart illustrating process used by Yassa et al. (1990) to select subjects for a study of tardive dyskinesia in schizophrenics with a history of neuroleptic use.

MEASURING PAST EXPOSURE

Causes of psychiatric illness are multifactorial and interactive, as described in Chapter 1. Etiologic agents may be biological, pharmacological, psychological, behavioral, or environmental (physical or social factors in the environment). Sources of exposure data include questionnaires, written records, and biomarkers. Questionnaires depend upon memory retrieval of a past exposure and may be administered face to face, over the telephone, or by mail. Face-to-face interviews provide the maximum flexibility, but subjects may refuse to travel to the interview or to allow interviews at home. Telephone interviews are quicker and cheaper than face-to-face interviews but are unsuitable for complex questionnaires or use of visual aids. In addition, some subjects may be reluctant to answer questions on the telephone due to the recent intrusion of telemarketing. Mailed questionnaires are the least expensive but have the poorest response rates (usually less than 50%). Regardless of mode of administration, questionnaires should be pilot-tested and standardized, and raters should not know whether the subject is a case or control.

Written records of medical, environmental, or occupational exposures provide an inexpensive and objective means for determining exposure status and are often the only source of exposure information which predates a disease. Unfortunately, records of exposures may be inaccurate, unavailable, or incomplete, as in the case study example. Accordingly, investigators should take special care in the design and testing of their record abstraction form (such as a form to determine previous dosage and duration of neuroleptic use), training and supervision of abstractors, scaling of exposure variables, and treatment of missing data (such as gaps in medication records). Availability and completeness of recorded exposure data should not differ between cases or controls.

Exposures have multiple dimensions which are rarely exploited for the information they might yield. Most case-control studies cite presence or absence of an exposure. However, exposures occur on varying levels of intensity, duration, accumulation, average exposure, peak exposure, time since first exposure, and time since last exposure. While exposure to antipsychotic drugs is an excellent example of the multiple dimensions of exposure, other typical exposures such as environmental stressors also have varied qualitative and quantitative properties. (See Chapter 1 for discussion of the quantitative properties of stressful life events.) Assessing multiple dimensions of an exposure allows for more different kinds of estimates of effects. Yassa and colleagues identified a variety of exposure factors measured in multiple dimensions: (1) age of onset of psychosis, (2) age at initiation of neuroleptic treatment, (3) total intake of psychotropic drugs, (4) *DSM-III* diagnosis, (5) organic conditions, (6) drug-free periods (months), and (7) when the movement disorder was first noted in the chart.

Strategies for the optimal measurement of exposures are listed in Table 8–8.

TABLE 8–8. Common strategies when measuring exposure

- Define explicitly all relevant exposure variables
- Choose exposure variable based on specific etiologic hypotheses
- Measure multiple dimensions of exposure, both current and past
- Identify which component of exposure is expected to operate at which point in the natural history of the disease
- Blind those who are measuring exposure status to the disorder status
- Use comparable methods of exposure measurement for both cases and controls
- Test the comparability among cases and controls of response rates on all measures of exposure
- Measure the prevalence of extraneous variables which may be related to exposure status or response rates

QUANTIFYING THE ODDS OF AN EXPOSURE FOR A GIVEN DISORDER

Once the exposure and disorder status are determined for each member of the sample, the magnitude of the association between the exposure and the disorder is assessed by comparing the odds of having been exposed among cases and controls. When the exposure and disorder status each have two levels, dividing the odds of being exposed among new cases by the odds of being exposed among noncases yields the *exposure odds ratio*. This estimated odds ratio by itself is not informative about the degree to which chance may have affected the measure of association. The confidence interval provides this information. In studies using unbiased samples from two populations of cases and controls, repeated trials should yield estimates of the exposure odds ratio which fall, with a specific level of dependability (such as 95% or 99%), within the calculated *confidence interval*. In case-control studies, the odds ratio and confidence interval is calculated as shown in Table 8–9.

The frequencies of various exposure factors among cases and controls in the case example are shown in Table 8–10. Note that the results suggest that mental retardation was the only organic condition for which the odds of occurrence differed among cases and controls. The statistical difference in the odds was tested with a chi-square statistic (cf. Chapter 12), but neither an odds ratio nor a confidence interval was calculated. This is easily done, and, in fact, calculating such estimates yields additional information over and above that provided by a test of statistical significance, particularly for exposure factors which are not statistically significant. For example, the odds of a history of insulin coma were not statistically different in the two groups. But one might like to know the magnitude and direction of the association between insulin coma and moderate-to-severe TD as well as how great the point estimate might be in other unbiased samples. The calculations from Table 8–11 are as follows:

$$\text{Exposure odds ratio} = (8 \times 54) / (12 \times 81) = .44$$

TABLE 8–9. Case-control studies: sample 2×2 cross-tabulation table and calculation of exposure odds ratio (OR_E) and confidence interval (CI)

	CASES	CONTROLS	
EXPOSED	a	b	$a + b$
UNEXPOSED	c	d	$c + d$
	$a + c$	$b + d$	$a + b + c + d$

$$\text{Exposure odds ratio } (OR_E) = \left(\frac{a/(a+c)}{c/(a+c)} \right) \div \left(\frac{b/(b+d)}{d/(b+d)} \right) = \frac{(a \times d)}{(b \times c)}$$

$$\text{Confidence interval } (CI) = \exp \left\{ \ln(OR_E) \pm \left(x \times \sqrt{\frac{1}{a} + \frac{1}{b} + \frac{1}{c} + \frac{1}{d}} \right) \right\}$$

where x = standard deviation of the normal curve for
% confidence desired (1.96 for 95% CI and 2.58 for 99% CI)

TABLE 8–10. Organic factors and treatments in 155 patients with moderate-to-severe or mild tardive dyskinesia

FACTOR OR TREATMENT	PATIENTS WITH MODERATE-TO-SEVERE TARDIVE DYSKINESIA ($n = 89$)		PATIENTS WITH MILD TARDIVE DYSKINESIA ($n = 66$)	
	n	%	n	%
Diabetes mellitus	14	15.7	9	13.6
Insulin coma	8	9.0	12	18.2
ECT	24	27.0	25	37.9
Cardiovascular disease	19	21.3	14	21.2
Mental retardation[a]	15	16.9	2	3.0

[a]Significantly more patients with moderate-to-severe tardive dyskinesia had this factor ($\chi^2 = 7.4$, df = 1, p < .001)
Data from Yassa et al., 1990

TABLE 8–11. Derived 2 × 2 cross-tabulation table for insulin coma treatment

	CASES (Moderate-to-Severe TD)	CONTROLS (Mild TD)	
EXPOSED	8 (9%)	12 (18%)	20
UNEXPOSED	81 (91%)	54 (82%)	135
	89	**66**	155

Data from Yassa et al., 1990

The standard error of that estimate is:

$$\sqrt{(1/8 + 1/12 + 1/81 + 1/54)}, \text{ or } .489$$

The upper and lower 95% confidence boundaries are, respectively:

$$\exp\{\ln(.44) + [1.96 \times .489]\}, \text{ or } 1.16$$

and

$$\exp\{\ln(.44) - [1.96 \times .489]\}, \text{ or } 0.17$$

In other words, the ratio of the odds of a history of insulin coma treatment among severe-to-moderate TD patients compared to the odds of a history of insulin coma treatment among mild TD patients was .44 to 1.00. Also, there was sufficient variability in the sample that the ratio of the two odds may have been as low as .17 to 1.00 or as high as 1.16 to 1.00.

Calculating the exposure odds ratio with confidence intervals gives the reader much more information about the association of exposure and disorder than is available from simple proportions. Specifically, it tells the reader the estimated magnitude of the ratio of the two exposure probabilities and how widely that estimate might range if multiple samples of TD patients were studied. It can be concluded from the calculations that although a history of insulin coma treatment appears to be protective against the more severe forms of TD (i.e., reduced odds of this treatment among severe TD patients by more than half), chance alone could have produced a ratio of that magnitude. Furthermore, there was enough variability in the cited study such that the odds of a positive history of insulin coma treatment could be as much as 16% higher among moderate-to-severe TD patients. Having an estimate of the magnitude of the protective effect and the potential variability of that estimate provides clinicians and investigators with a benchmark against which to compare other risk factors as well as to assess the comparability of their patient populations to the study population.

In the case example, the authors also collected data on a variety of exposure variables which were scaled continuously. Their primary analytic strategy with these factors was to compare mean exposure levels between pairs of outcome groups (mild vs. moderate, mild vs. severe, and moderate vs. severe) and to test with a t-statistic the likelihood that differences in means of a given magnitude could have occurred by chance (cf. Chapter 12). An alternative strategy for exposures measured on an ordinal or continuous scale is to rescale them into discrete categories based on scientifically sound, clinically meaningful dosage levels and/or the frequency distribution of the exposure across the entire study sample, e.g., interquartile ranges. When an exposure variable has more than two levels, the exposure odds ratio reflects the increasing (or decreasing) magnitude of risk for each increment (or reduction) in dosage level of the exposure.

To estimate the effect of multiple exposures on the presence or absence of a psychiatric disorder, researchers often use *logistic regression* modeling procedures (see Chapter 12). Adjusting the exposure odds of one exposure variable for the presence of other related factors optimizes the use of case-control data. Yassa et al. found in their study that the simple (unadjusted) probability of mental retardation was significantly greater in patients with moderate-to-severe TD than in those with mild TD. But this relationship may be spurious if other variables, such as long-term exposure to psychotropic medications prescribed in the context of a neurologic condition such as mental retardation, are confounding the supposed association. A model that included both the organic condition and other parameters of psychotropic drug history would have been more useful to consumers of clinical research for understanding the most precise, unconfounded estimates of exposure odds.

Problem Set

Brown and Birley (1968) studied how interpersonal relationships affect the course of schizophrenia, assessing stressful life events in detail. The study hypothesis, based on pilot research, was that "first and subsequent acute schizophrenic attacks were . . . produced . . . by crises and life changes . . . in the three weeks before the attack" (Brown and Birley, 1968, p. 203).

Case notes on all patients newly admitted to hospitals serving a population of 1,000,000 in England were reviewed for evidence of schizophrenia. Potential cases were examined by one of two psychiatrists and diagnosed using conventional Kraepelinian criteria. Subjects included the first 50 cases identified as meeting the following criteria: (1) first or recurrent onset of psychotic symptoms could be dated within a 1-week span and occurred within the 12 weeks prior to admission, and (2) subject was diagnosed as schizophrenic or having schizoaffective or mixed affective disorder with paranoid ideas.

To construct a control group, an invitation to participate in a medical research project was sent to a random sample of employees of six local firms, all of whom were clerical workers, building laborers, or skilled, semiskilled, or unskilled factory workers. Ninety-five percent ($n = 377$) of the employees agreed to be interviewed at their place of work. Fifty-two employees identified as "foreign or West Indian" were excluded because such subjects were not represented in the case group.

Both groups were administered a scale measuring stressful life events which had been developed by the researchers. Events involved the subjects themselves or a close relative. Possible events were those which on the grounds of common sense were likely to produce emotional disturbance in many people, including changes in roles, health, residence or amount of social interaction, the forecast of such change, or the fulfillment or disappointment of a goal. The exposure variable (events) was categorized in three levels: "independent events . . . imposed on the subject and outside his control"; "possibly independent events . . . for which the claim of independence was

TABLE 8–12. Percentage of persons experiencing at least one life event in each of the four 3-week periods before onset (patients, $n = 50$) or interview (general population, $n = 325$)

	PERCENTAGE OF RESPONDENTS REPORTING STRESSFUL LIFE EVENTS IN EACH 3-WEEK PERIOD BEFORE ONSET OR INTERVIEW			
	(FURTHEST) 4TH[a] (%)	3RD[a] (%)	2ND[a] (%)	(NEAREST) 1ST[b] (%)
Patients	30	18	20	60
General population	21	20	18	19

[a] Comparisons not significant ($p > .05$) for other periods

[b] For the first 3-week period, $p < .001$ (two-tailed χ^2 test with 1 df)

Data from Brown and Birley, 1968

likely but not assumed"; and "no event" for all subjects who reported no stressful life events of the types described in the prior 3 months (p. 205).

Face-to-face interviews were conducted with controls at their place of employment and with patients and relatives at an unspecified place. Patients and relatives were interviewed separately by one of two psychiatrists, and events were rated independently.

The case and control groups did not differ with respect to age, gender, nationality, or education. Cases were less likely to be married, more likely to live alone or with parents, and less likely to have seen other relatives in the past year. The main results of the study are displayed in Table 8–12.

The authors concluded that "there is reasonably sound evidence that environmental factors can precipitate a schizophrenic attack and that such events tend to cluster in the 3 weeks before onset" (p. 211). Caveats included the possibility of interviewer contamination (since both psychiatrists were aware of the hypothesis) and of events having precipitated the admission rather than the onset of symptoms.

Questions

1. Is a case-control design appropriate to the aim of this study?

2. What advantages and disadvantages attend the source population for these cases? How representative of all schizophrenia patients is the source population?

3. What alternative source(s) for cases could be used?

4. Are cases incident or prevalent cases? Is this a problem? If so, why?

5. What is the source population for the controls, and what are the criteria for inclusion as a "control"? In what ways are criteria for selection as a control similar to and different from criteria for selection as a case? What are the advantages and disadvantages of this source of controls? How likely is it that this source of controls will include undetected cases of schizophrenia (false negatives)?

6. What other source(s) could be used?

7. What are the advantages and disadvantages of face-to-face interviews for measuring stressful life events?

8. What alternative method for measurement of exposure status might be used, and with what advantages and disadvantages?

9. Using the data from Table 8–12, compare the probability of stressful life events (SLE) in the nearest 3-week period to onset or interview (O/I) with the respective probabilities of such events in the 2nd, 3rd, and 4th periods. Fill in the blank 2 × 2 tables in Table 8–13 with cell frequencies for patients and controls and calculate for each period the odds ratios and confidence intervals comparing exposure rates in the two groups for past stressful life events.

10. State in words the exposure odds ratios and confidence intervals for each period of exposure.

11. What is the range of estimates of three-week period prevalence of any stressful life event among controls in this study? What is the range of comparable estimates for cases?

12. Explain the sources of bias which could plausibly be operating in this study based on your experience with taking histories from schizophrenic patients.

TABLE 8–13. Blank 2×2 tables for question 9

PERSONS EXPERIENCING AT LEAST ONE STRESSFUL LIFE EVENT (SLE) DURING:

a) Nearest (1st) period:
   0–3 weeks before O/I

	Cases	Controls
SLE		
No SLE		

b) 2nd period:
   4–6 weeks before O/I

	Cases	Controls
SLE		
No SLE		

c) 3rd period:
   7–9 weeks before O/I

	Cases	Controls
SLE		
No SLE		

d) 4th period:
   10–12 weeks before O/I

	Cases	Controls
SLE		
No SLE		

13. Give one alternative explanation of the findings reported by these authors, and briefly describe the type of study which could test your hypothesis.

Answers

1. Yes. Schizophrenia is rare in the community. Affected persons usually come to the attention of medical personnel. Stressful life events (SLE) are common although eliciting information about these events is a time-consuming interview process using the methods of these investigators. The investigators minimized time, effort, and expense by using a methodology which maximized the availability of treated schizophrenics and compared their SLE rates to the rates among "typical" community persons.

2. Sampling all hospitals in a geographic area insured the representativeness of hospitalized cases in an entire community population, and hospitalized patients are certainly more accessible than outpatients or currently untreated persons. However, if onset of psychiatric symptoms did not universally result in hospitalization, and the decision not to hospitalize was related to the level of stress in the home, then the exposure history of the case group may not be representative of that for all schizophrenic patients. Furthermore, this case group is likely to include more severe cases and fewer chronic cases. Persons with poor support in the home may also be overrepresented as cases regardless of the frequency of stressful life events associated with hospitalization for a psychotic episode.

3. Including outpatients would provide a more complete range of presentations of this disease in the sample, and one could test the role of confounding posed by hospitalization with this larger source of cases. However, the logistic difficulties of identifying, sampling, and interviewing such a population of patients would be considerable.

4. By including patients with onset of either first or recurrent symptoms, the investigators have assembled prevalent cases. Varying degrees of disease chronicity or treatment history may confound the association of stressful life events and symptom onset in such a case group. For example, recurrent cases may be more likely to be hospitalized than incident cases.

5. Controls were blue-collar and office workers from England who were willing to participate. Criteria for selection of the local firms were not explained nor were comparisons (beyond education) made between controls and cases. It seems unlikely that these clerical and manual laborers would be as representative of the entire population of 1,000,000 persons as would cases from all hospitals serving that community. This control group had a high response rate, but it underrepresented professionals, homemakers, the self-employed, retirees, and the unemployed. As the authors point out, life crises have been shown to be more prevalent among the disadvantaged, and therefore employed controls may be less likely than the unemployed to report such crises. Although it is unlikely that an em-

ployed person could undergo a completely undetected acute schizophrenic episode (given its accompanying dysfunction), a thorough screening of this control group should include data on any history of psychiatric help-seeking or hospitalization or use of psychiatric medication in order to eliminate controls with a past history of disorders associated with SLE.

6. Multiple control groups of unaffected persons from other care sites and various socioeconomic strata would help dispel concerns about dissimilarities between cases and controls. Such groups might include psychiatric patients with other (nonschizophrenic) disorders for which SLE have not been implicated as risk or prognostic factors, schizophrenic patients in outpatient care, neighbors of cases, or a group selected by random-digit dialing. Multiple comparisons provide useful information about which biases are most germane to an observed association.

7. Face-to-face interviews provide the opportunity to explore the qualitative nature of stressful life events and the dating of events using intricate probes necessary for retrospective recall. However, this SLE questionnaire takes 1–3 hours to complete, which is particularly burdensome for patients but also for controls. Face-to-face interviews can also be subject to bias, especially where the interviewers are not blinded to case status. Although it might be difficult to blind interviewers to schizophrenia status, they might easily be blinded to the study hypothesis, diminishing the chance that an interviewer would probe for near-term events among cases. Categorizing subjects with respect to exposure status (independent events, possibly independent events, and no events) could be accomplished by personnel blinded to both case status and study hypotheses.

8. Telephone interviews would provide the advantages of reduced costs and possibly shorter total time per subject. However, patients, in particular, would likely not tolerate a telephone interview as well as a face-to-face encounter. Mailed questionnaires also provide notoriously low response rates, particularly among controls who may feel little obligation to take nonwork time to complete such an instrument; mail surveys would be especially inappropriate for the SLE scaling procedures used by Brown and colleagues.

9. Cross-tabulation tables are shown in Table 8–14. (Data from Table 8–12 are shown in boldface).

10. Patients hospitalized for acute onset of psychotic symptoms were more than six times as likely to have experienced a stressful life event in the 3 weeks prior to the onset of symptoms than were employed persons in the 3 weeks prior to being interviewed. Repeated samples for the same populations could show differences of as little as 3.39 times the likelihood or as much as 11.95 times the likelihood of a stressful life event. The patient group had 1.13, .88, and 1.62 times the odds of a stressful life event in the 4–6-, 7–9-, and 10–12-week periods prior to onset of symptoms, respectively, compared to the same periods of time prior to the interview for the control group, but ratios of these magnitudes could have occurred by chance and the odds may in truth be even (1.00).

TABLE 8–14. 2×2 cross-tabulation tables, with odds ratios and confidence intervals

(a) Experienced at least 1 stress event during nearest (1st) period
    (0–3 weeks before onset or interview)

	Cases	Controls		Odds Ratio *(Confidence Interval)*
Stress Event	30 (**60%**)	62 (**19%**)	92	6.36 *(3.39, 11.95)*
No Stress Event	20	263	283	
	50	**325**	375	

(b) Experienced at least 1 stress event during 2nd period
    (4–6 weeks before onset or interview)

	Cases	Controls		Odds Ratio *(Confidence Interval)*
Stress Event	10 (**20%**)	59 (**18%**)	69	1.13 *(0.53, 2.38)*
No Stress Event	40	266	306	
	50	**325**	375	

(c) Experienced at least 1 stress event during 3rd period
    (7–9 weeks before onset or interview)

	Cases	Controls		Odds Ratio *(Confidence Interval)*
Stress Event	9 (**18%**)	65 (**20%**)	74	0.88 *(0.41, 1.90)*
No Stress Event	41	260	301	
	50	**325**	375	

continued

TABLE 8–14. *(Continued)*

(d) Experienced at least 1 stress event during 4th period
(10–12 weeks before onset or interview)

	Cases	Controls		Odds Ratio *(Confidence Interval)*
Stress Event	15 (**30%**)	68 (**21%**)	83	1.62 *(0.84, 3.14)*
No Stress Event	35	257	292	
	50	**325**	375	

Based on data from Brown and Birley, 1968

11. The control group demonstrated an estimated 3-week-period prevalence for SLE of 18–21%. The 3-week prevalence for cases was similar (18–30%) during the weeks which were more distant from the interview.

12. The authors addressed three serious biases in "stress" research: effort after meaning, interviewer effects, and the mixing of cause and effect. Effort after meaning refers to the tendency of human subjects (usually cases) to exaggerate, or even simply to remember events differently, as a way of explaining a disorder or other outcome. To counter this bias, the authors constructed a list of event probes to equalize the different salience of events among patients and controls. Rates of event occurrence were similar among cases and controls except in the 3 weeks prior to onset, suggesting that cases were not more likely than controls to remember events within the more distant 12-week recall period.

Interviewer effects might occur if the interviewers probed for recent events among cases but not among controls. The authors note that most events were major ones and easily dated and that independently assessed data from cases and their relatives compared favorably.

The most serious bias attends all cross-sectional and retrospective designs, and that involves the mixing of exposure and outcome. Particularly in this example, where the prognostic impact of crises and life changes on course of illness was being explored, the fact of a preexisting illness, especially of the socially disruptive nature of schizophrenia, must be considered as the possible direct or indirect cause, as well as a possible outcome, of stressful life events. One might well argue that a number of the "independent" event-exposures (including the hospitalization of family members for physical or mental illness; arrest of family members for criminal behavior; job changes; physical deterioration and/or hospitalization of living partners; participation as witness or judgments against the subject in a lawsuit; discontinuing education; and diagnosis of serious infection) might be caused indirectly or directly by a history of a severe mental disorder such as schizophrenia in a family member. Many of these events categorized as "independent" seem, at best, "possibly independent," and the authors provided no operational definitions adequate to the task of discriminating between exposure levels.

13. A competing explanation for this finding would be that the burden of schizophrenic symptomatology plays a role in many of the crises and life changes mentioned by the patient and his or her social network, including all those related to increases in felt distress, compromised immune systems, and adaptive and maladaptive changes in the patient's social environment.

One methodologic strategy for testing this alternative would be to enroll incident cases only. Then one could be assured that the first overt symptoms of the disease occurred following the events (although it could be argued that prodromal symptoms might trigger such events). Although the authors tested the association between events and symptom onset separately for prevalent ($n = 31$) and incident ($n = 19$) cases and found an elevation in near-term events in both groups, the sample sizes were small, and statistical tests may well have been unstable.

Alternatively, in a prospective study of relapse only, the investigators might begin with a symptom-free sample of schizophrenic patients and measure exposure (events) and outcome (symptom onset) prospectively and repeatedly over a period of months, as well as measuring potential confounders such as social support and other factors related to course. If they hypothesized that the base rate of crises and life events among the unaffected population was approximately 14%, then the follow-up period would need to be long enough to accrue an adequate number of exposed subjects. At the end of the study, occurrence of any crisis or life event in specified time periods would determine exposure status. Such a follow-up study would decrease selection and recall bias, but with greater expense, greater respondent burden, and with likely increases in losses to follow-up, especially among controls.

REFERENCES

Bauer M.S., Calabrese J., Dunner D.L., Post R., Whybrow P.C., Gyulai L., Tay L.K., Younkin S.R., Bynum D., Lavori P., Price R.A. 1994. Multisite data reanalysis of the validity of rapid cycling as a course modifier for bipolar disorder in DSM-IV. *American Journal of Psychiatry* 151: 506–515.

Brown G.W., Birley J.L.T. 1968. Crises and life changes and the onset of schizophrenia. *Journal of Health and Social Behavior* 9: 203–214.

Gail M., Williams R., Byar D.P., Brown C. 1976. How many controls? *Journal of Chronic Diseases* 29: 723–731.

Guth C., Jones P., Murray R. 1993. Familial psychiatric illness and obstetric complications in early-onset affective disorder. A case-control study. *British Journal of Psychiatry* 163: 492–498.

Hickie I., Hickie C., Lloyd A., Silove D., Wakefield D. 1993. Impaired in vivo immune responses in patients with melancholia. *British Journal of Psychiatry* 162: 651–657.

Holroyd S., Rabins P.V., Finkelstein D., Nicholson M.C., Chase G.A., Wisniewski S.C. 1992. Visual hallucinations in patients with macular degeneration. *American Journal of Psychiatry* 149: 1701–1706.

Lesage A.D., Boyer R., Grunberg F., Vanier C., Morissette R., Menard-Buteau C., Loyer M. 1994. Suicide and mental disorders: a case-control study of young men. *American Journal of Psychiatry* 151: 1063–1068.

Rothman K.J. 1986. *Modern Epidemiology.* New York: Little, Brown.

Simpson G.M., Lee H.J., Zoubak B., Gardos G.L. 1979. A rating scale for tardive dyskinesia. *Psychopharmacology* 64: 171–179.

U.S. National Institute of Mental Health (US-NIMH). 1975. *Development of a Dyskinetic Movement Scale* (Publ. No. 4). Rockville, MD: National Institute of Mental Health, Psychopharmacology Research Branch.

Welch S.L., Fairburn C.G. 1994. Sexual abuse and bulimia nervosa: three integrated case control comparisons. *American Journal of Psychiatry* 151: 402–407.

Wessely S., Castle D., Der G., Murray R. 1991. Schizophrenia and Afro-Caribbeans: a case-control study. *British Journal of Psychiatry* 159: 795–801.

Winsa B., Adami H.-O., Bergstrom R., Gamstedt A., Dahlberg P.A., Adamson U., Jansson R., Karlsson A. 1991. Stressful life events and Graves' disease. *Lancet* 338: 1475–1479.

Yassa R., Nair N.P.V., Iskandar H., Schwartz G. 1990. Factors in the development of severe forms of tardive dyskinesia. *American Journal of Psychiatry* 147: 1156–1163.

Zametkin A.J., Liebenauer L.L., Fitzgerald G.A., King A.C., Minkunas D.V., Herscovitch P., Yamada E.M., Cohen R.M. 1993. Brain metabolism in teenagers with attention-deficit hyperactivity disorder. *Archives of General Psychiatry* 50: 333–340.

9

CLINICAL TRIALS

OBJECTIVES

- To describe the goals of clinical trials: primary, secondary, and tertiary prevention.
- To review the ethical and practical problems associated with clinical trials.
- To describe the methods of a typical clinical trial.
- To review the procedures used by the pharmaceutical industry when bringing a newly discovered compound to market as a medication.

CASE EXAMPLE

In 1994, a group of investigators explored the relative effectiveness of the selective serotonin reuptake inhibitor (SSRI) fluoxetine compared to the tricyclic antidepressant (TCA) nortriptyline in 64 older adults experiencing comorbid major depression and cardiovascular disease. They randomly assigned subjects to receive either fluoxetine or nortriptylene and followed them for two weeks to determine both the effectiveness of treatment. The investigators concluded from this single-blind study that fluoxetine was significantly less effective than nortriptyline in treating hospitalized elderly patients with unipolar major depression, especially those with the melancholic subtype and concurrent cardiovascular disease (Roose et al., 1994).

INTRODUCTION

The clinical trial, which involves the direct comparison of two or more interventions (one of which may be no actual in human groups, is the core method for studying the effectiveness of drugs and other treatments for psychiatric disorders. The goal of a clinical trial is to test the efficacy, or relative efficacy, of a therapeutic or preventive agent or technique.

Clinical trials include a wide range of studies, but in psychiatry they are studies of interventions directed at the onset, chronicity, or effects of psychiatric disorders. For example, a clinical trial designed as a community-based study may focus on the effectiveness of behavioral interventions vs. other interventions in reducing the frequency of smoking. The hoped-for outcome is smoking reduction and a decrease in smoking-related physical and psychiatric disorders. Such a study explores different ways of achieving prevention (smoking cessation) of a disorder (lung cancer). Such studies are called studies of primary prevention. In primary prevention, the disorder is prevented from occurring in the first place.

Clinical trials may also be used to test a medication or form of psychotherapy to reverse the symptoms of a psychiatric disorder, such as major depression, that has recently developed. These studies are called studies of secondary prevention— i.e., early remission of a disorder. Clinical trials are also carried out to study efforts to reduce disability secondary to an advanced disorder. For instance, the relative effectiveness of two antipsychotic medications, such as clozapine and haloperidol, in reducing disability from schizophrenia might be compared in a clinical trial. The reduction of disabilities due to a chronic illness is referred to as tertiary prevention.

PROTECTION OF HUMAN SUBJECTS

Before beginning a clinical trial, an investigator must address certain issues. The most important are ethical issues. The federal government requires that each institution (such as a hospital or clinic in which clinical trials are performed) review the ethical implications of trials by an Institutional Review Board (IRB). This board must determine that the research design is ethical given our current understanding of therapy for a given disease. Specifically, the IRB must determine if the benefits of the trial are greater than the potential harm to subjects, that subjects will

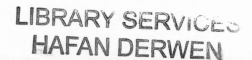

be adequately informed, and that the methods of the trial are likely to produce results which are useful and can be generalized. In the Roose et al. (1994) study, the investigators were required to convince the IRB of the New York State Psychiatric Institute that sufficient questions remained unanswered regarding the relative efficacy of fluoxetine vs. nortriptyline to warrant a clinical trial. The investigators were also required to demonstrate that the risk-to-benefit ratio warranted the trial. Because all patients received a medication and because antidepressant therapy is considered an appropriate therapy for major depression, the investigators should have encountered little difficulty convincing the IRB that the benefit of antidepressant therapy was greater than the risk. Because both drugs are used in the medically ill elderly, the rationale for the trial was straightforward. Investigators in clinical trials must address other ethical questions as well.

Is the Proposed Treatment a Safe Treatment?

Both fluoxetine and nortriptyline have been proven relatively safe drugs in therapy of medically ill, depressed, older adults. Yet patients with cardiovascular disease have been thought to be at increased risk for side effects with TCAs, although this is a much-debated topic.

Does the Study Design Deny Treatment to Persons When Some Form of Treatment Is Known to Be of Benefit?

In this case, no subject was denied treatment (except for a 2-week "washout period" before treatment assignment). If the results were dramatic, the investigators would have to determine if they should stop the treatment and make the more effective therapy available to everyone. In the Roose et al. study, although the investigators found a significant difference in favor of nortriptyline, the difference was not dramatic, and there was no reason during the study to stop the study and switch all participants to nortriptyline.

Should Subjects Be Denied Participation in the Clinical Trial?

Subjects in the Roose et al. study were required to meet inclusion criteria (described below). Subjects excluded from the trial were not excluded from receiving one of the existing therapies if considered clinically efficacious. The investigators would be open to criticism for denying therapy if they were testing a new drug not currently available in clinical practice but which had been found extremely effective in preliminary trials—much more effective and/or more safe than existing therapies for depression in medically ill, older adults.

Finally, the IRB must be convinced that the subjects in a trial are adequately informed of the nature of the trial and the risks vs. benefits. The IRB will carefully review the consent form to be signed by each subject. As many clinical trials have been instituted over the years, a new investigator should never attempt to devise a consent form "from scratch." Forms from other trials should be used as templates.

Feasibility

Once ethical issues are addressed, the feasibility of a particular research design must be addressed. In the "best of all possible worlds," an investigator or pharmaceutical company would wish to test a new antidepressant agent against a placebo, for then a clear difference might be determined. Yet, a medically ill, depressed, older adult may not be permitted by his or her attending physician to be given a placebo. In many studies, to test the effectiveness of a new antidepressant, the new drug is compared to imipramine (the gold standard of antidepressant therapy). If the drug is equivalent to imipramine in efficacy, the drug may be compared to imipramine for side effects.

Next, the investigators must determine whether enough subjects can be recruited to demonstrate a difference in the therapies compared. As with other research designs, investigators can only generalize their results to a population from which their sample is drawn. The goal of the study by Roose and colleagues was to compare two antidepressant agents in older persons with a combination of severe depression and medical illness. Some evidence (though far from conclusive) existed prior to the study that SSRIs were less effective than tricyclic antidepressants in treating patients with the melancholic subtype of major depression. Investigators also had an interest in the cardiovascular effects of antidepressant agents in patients with cardiovascular disease comorbid with major depression, a not uncommon presentation of depression among older adults. These investigators therefore had to determine whether they could recruit enough subjects who met their inclusion and exclusion criteria to demonstrate a difference between fluoxetine and nortriptyline in medically ill older adults. As they had no guidelines, they could not perform a power analysis, i.e., an analysis to determine the number of subjects needed to demonstrate a difference in efficacy of statistical significance (see below). Therefore, they assumed that 64 patients would be sufficient to find a difference in the two antidepressant agents in efficacy. Sixty-four subjects is a moderate-sized sample for a clinical trial and is a reasonable estimate of the number of subjects the investigators could recruit. Yet these investigators must have realized that they could only hope to have selected a reasonable sample size.

How do investigators decide the size of a sample which will demonstrate a statistically significant difference between the treatment and the control group? There are formulas to determine how large a sample is needed (formulas not only applicable to clinical trials but other types of studies as well). The application of the formulas to determine an adequate sample size is often called a power analysis.

The investigator must know or make an educated guess about the following information in order to use one of these formulas in order to determine sample size:

- The Type I error willing to be accepted (See Chapter 12)
- The Type II error willing to be accepted (See Chapter 12)
- The difference between the control and treatment groups on a measure which is accepted as a meaningful difference (e.g., the difference between the control and treatment groups on the HDRS)
- The mean and standard deviation of the measure (e.g., HDRS) in the population sample. Examples of these formulas can be found in most statistics textbooks.

Finally, the cost of a clinical trial must be taken into account. The vast majority of clinical trials are funded by pharmaceutical companies. For many years, pharmaceutical companies would pay an investigator "up front" with the assumption that the investigator could recruit a certain number of subjects into the study and complete the protocol with those subjects. During recent, more difficult economic times pharmaceutical companies have changed, in large part, their orientation toward funding clinical trials. They still provide some dollars "up front," but they then pay investigators a predetermined amount for each subject who completes the study. For a typical trial, for example, comparing a new antidepressant agent to an existing agent, a company may pay up to $3,000–4,000 per subject who completes the trial. As monies must be targeted for advertising, for maintaining a clinical coordinator (even when subject flow is slow), and for the lack of reimbursement for subjects who do not complete the study, this amount is not excessive. Investigators must therefore, given past experience, determine if they can afford financially to participate in a clinical trial sponsored by a pharmaceutical company. Some clinical trials are funded through the National Institutes of Health and foundations, but once again, the investigator must be able to estimate the cost of recruiting and completing the study with the desired number of subjects when preparing the budget of the grant proposal. Some studies, such as the Roose study, are funded internally by state or federal institutions, such as the New York Psychiatric Institute or the Veterans Administration, as part of an overall "research allocation" from state or federal agencies to that institution.

RESEARCH DESIGN—STATING THE HYPOTHESIS

Investigators should state, a priori, a clear hypothesis which includes a definition of a "case," a "control," and a clear definition of the desired end point and how that end point is to be measured. In particular, investigators should define meaningful improvement (or a meaningful difference between treatments).

In the Roose study, older adults (average age of 73 years) with a diagnosis of cardiac disease, major depression with melancholia, and a Hamilton Depression Rating Scale (HDRS) score of 18 or greater who had completed a 2-week place- bo "washout" were the subjects included. Cardiac disease required that the sub- jects have impaired left ventricular function which was defined by an injection fraction of 50% or less, a ventricular arrhythmia, conduction disease, or a combi- nation of these conditions. Subjects who had been successfully treated or who had been treated with medications that met standards of minimal adequacy, such as imipramine 150 mg a day for 2 weeks, were excluded. Subjects were defined as responders to the drug to which they were randomly assigned (1) if they reported return to baseline functioning, that is, function before the beginning of the de- pressive episode, or (2) if they were able to leave the hospital for 2 weeks without requiring adjustment in dose of the medication and the final HDRS score was less than 8. Though not stated, the implicit null hypothesis was that older adults with major depression with melancholia and cardiovascular disease would respond equally well to the TCA nortriptyline and the SSRI fluoxetine. The alternate hy- pothesis was that subjects would respond significantly better to nortriptyline than fluoxetine.

RESEARCH DESIGN

The basic design of a clinical trial is presented in Figure 9–1. In the Roose study, the reference population included older, hospitalized, depressed patients with car- diovascular disease. The experimental population included all inpatients at the New York State Psychiatric Institute who met the inclusion and exclusion criteria. Sixty-four of these patients became subjects in the study, i.e., the study sample.

The investigators could have selected the participants in a number of ways, such as advertising for volunteer subjects or even making participation in the study a requisite for receiving a given therapy (usually an experimental therapy not gen- erally available). In this case, however, the investigators selected subjects who were admitted to the hospital and offered them an opportunity to participate in the study—i.e., they used a convenience sample. Once selected to enter the study, sub- jects were "randomly assigned" to either fluoxetine or nortriptyline treatment. In this study, design was varied from usual patterns in that more subjects were as- signed to the nortriptyline than the fluoxetine group (42 vs. 22 subjects). Random assignment can be accomplished by using a random number table (a table which can be generated by computer) and utilizing numbers randomly generated by the computer to assign a subject to either of the two treatment groups.

Other approaches to assigning subjects to one group vs. another are less satis- factory, but are used. For example, paired sampling may be used. In this case, al- ternate cases are assigned randomly, and the "next case" is assigned to the oppo-

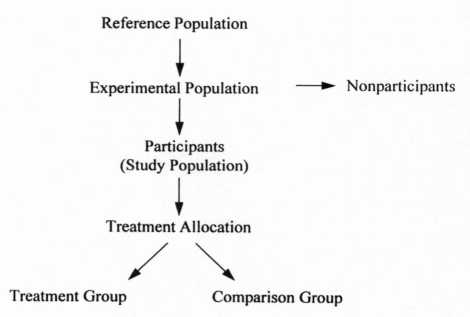

FIGURE 9–1. Basic design of a clinical trial.

site group. This ensures that the number of subjects in each group is equal or meets the exact proportion specified by the protocol. A much less satisfactory means of sampling is what is called "temporal cluster sampling." For example, all subjects attending a clinic during 1 month may be assigned to one treatment group and subjects attending the clinic the next month may be assigned to a different treatment group. These alternative assignment procedures do not distribute subjects as equally with respect to their other characteristics as does random assignment.

Types of "blinding" to assignment of treatment in clinical trials are presented in Table 9–1.

Most clinical trials are either double-blind or double-blind crossover studies. Occasionally there is no blinding and the trial is called an "open" trial. Another variant is a triple-blind study, in which the data analysts are blinded to results as well. The Roose study is a single-blind study: The investigators knew which drug

TABLE 9–1. Types of blinding to assignment of treatment in clinical trials

	KNOWLEDGE OF TREATMENT ASSIGNMENT	
Blinding	Patient	Investigator
None	Yes	Yes
Single	No	Yes
Double	No	No
Double-blind crossover	No	No

the subjects were receiving. If these investigators had a bias against fluoxetine, then the single-blind approach may not have been appropriate. For example, their perceptions that the nortriptyline subjects were doing better than the fluoxetine group may have affected their outcome measures, given that the HDRS requires a judgment on the part of the raters. In most cases, double-blind studies are much preferred. In a double-blind crossover study each patient receives both types of treatments (or receives a treatment for a part of the study and a placebo for another part of the study). However, long half-life of fluoxetine would render a double-blind crossover study difficult to perform with this patient population as it would require a second washout period of perhaps 2 weeks or longer.

The investigators must take care not to bias results, regardless of design, in terms of which subjects are included in the initial allocation. For example, if a criteria for participants in a study is tolerance for the medication, then individuals may be excluded initially from randomization because during the initial stage of examining the effects of a "test dose" of the drug, some subjects are eliminated because they cannot tolerate even one dose of the drug. If these subjects are eliminated, the trial is biased in favor of the drug being tested.

IMPLEMENTATION CHALLENGES

Once the study design is set, the investigator faces a new set of challenges. Recruitment of subjects to the study is a major challenge. As noted above, advertisements on radio, television, and in the printed press are frequently used recruiting strategies, encouraging persons exposed to reading the advertisement who have certain symptoms to call a telephone number to find out if they qualify for the study. Much time must be devoted to screening subjects who respond to the advertisement, and often the payoff is a tiny fraction of the initial volunteers.

Maintaining a high level of compliance in the study is another major challenge. Not only does low compliance increase the number of subjects the investigator must recruit to the study; low compliance also decreases the validity of whatever differences between treatment groups are found. In the Roose et al. study, of the 42 patients who received nortriptyline, 34 were able to complete the trial (4 weeks of drug compliance). Of the 22 patients randomly assigned to fluoxetine, 18 were able to complete the trial.

The determining a priori of an adequate period of follow-up in order to assess whether a medication is effective or not is another significant challenge. These investigators selected 4 weeks. For the study of antidepressive agents, beneficial effects usually appear within 4 weeks, but perhaps the full benefit of the drug cannot be observed until 5 or 6 weeks following initiation of therapy. On the other hand, the longer the duration of the study the higher the likelihood of noncompliance (that is, subjects will not complete the trial). Four weeks was an appropriate period of follow-up for the Roose study.

The selection of appropriate statistics to analyze the data a priori is yet another challenge. Simple statistical procedures can be used to compare treatment and control groups, yet many investigators use more complex statistics to take into account issues such as a difference in age, differences in diagnosis (albeit slight), and other factors. In the Roose study, the final conclusion that nortriptyline was a superior treatment to fluoxetine was based on a logistic regression analysis which controlled for the diagnosis of melancholia, age, and the HDRS prior to treatment (see Chapter 12).

RESULTS

The results of a clinical trial are usually straightforward. Every clinician using medications to treat a psychiatric disorder should learn to interpret the results of a clinical trial independently and not rely upon the conclusions presented by the authors of the study. For example, the results may demonstrate little difference between the treatment and control groups, yet the authors may conclude that the experimental treatment has been "proven" more effective and is therefore definitely to be preferred over the control treatment.

A LOOK INSIDE THE PHARMACEUTICAL INDUSTRY

In this country, most clinical trials for pharmaceutical agents are initiated by pharmaceutical companies. They, in turn, contract with academic health centers and other clinician-investigators to study medications which they have patented prior to testing those medications. The passage from discovery and development to marketing a new drug by a pharmaceutical company is generally conceived of as the "pipeline."

The first phase of the pipeline is the period of drug discovery. This discovery occurs in laboratories or through computer simulations and is outside the context of patient-oriented research. Hundreds and thousands of person-hours and millions of dollars are invested in discovering new compounds and bringing these compounds to the point where they can be studied in humans.

Once a compound is chosen and is elevated to "project status" (usually being assigned a code consisting of a combination of letters and numbers) the pharmaceutical company must receive permission from the Food and Drug Administration (FDA) to continue study of the compound. They must submit an application to the FDA indicating their desire to study the drug in humans. This application contains all of the preclinical data on the new compound, including reports on the synthesis, pharmacokinetics, pharmacodynamics, toxicology, biochemistry, chemical stability, and other data. The application also contains the protocol which is proposed by the company to be followed for the initial clinical study. Frequently, these compounds have been studied in other countries, and the results of these foreign studies are also included in the application. After this Investigational New Drug application (IND) is submitted, the FDA then must approve the IND in order for the pharmaceutical company to begin clinical studies.

Once the IND is approved, the drug is generally studied in three phases before the drug can be resubmitted to the FDA for a New Drug Application (NDA). Phase I studies are usually conducted in normal, healthy volunteers (in the past, usually males), who are paid to participate in these early studies. The previous bias against women derived from the fear that women might become pregnant during a clinical study, and therefore women were usually excluded even if they assured the company that they were not pregnant and had no plans to become pregnant.

There is an exception to using normal subjects for Phase I study: When it is known prior to beginning a Phase I study that the drug is expected to be toxic, subjects with the disease that the drug is hoped to successfully treat may be used. An example is clozapine, a drug that was known to cause agranulocytosis in a significant minority of persons taking the drug, but for which significant therapeutic benefits were thought to outweigh this potential toxic effect in refractory patients. In this case, the ethics of testing the new drug suggest that only persons who suffer from the disease be exposed to the drug.

From six to 20 volunteers usually receive one dose of the drug in Phase I of a study and then may receive a second dose 1 or 2 weeks after the first. The dose given is gradually increased, and a maximum safe daily dose level is established based upon both subjective report and objective examination of subjects. The major goal of Phase I studies is to prove the safety of the new drug in normal subjects and identify the tolerable dosage range. Pharmacokinetic data, such as the half-life of the drug, is also collected during this time through blood and urine samples. These data assist investigators in determining how frequently the drug must be administered. Phase I studies usually take about a year to complete.

Phase II studies are initiated to determine whether the drug is effective in treating the disorder for which it is targeted. Early Phase II studies usually include pilot studies with a few patients who have the disease or problems for which the drug is targeted. The simple question is, "Do patients improve who take the drug?" and therefore these are not controlled studies. If the drug shows promise, small, controlled clinical studies are performed on between 75 and 500 patients. Phase II studies may take between 2 and 5 years to complete and are frequently fraught with difficulties such as unexpected side effects and problems with drug absorption and metabolism. Many primary agents may not proceed beyond Phase II because of these side effects. If the drug proves successful during Phase II studies, then the pharmaceutical company sits down with the FDA to discuss the full NDA that the company will submit.

As the pharmaceutical company will invest millions of dollars during Phase III studies, they attempt to negotiate ahead of time with the FDA the specific types of studies, numbers of patients included, and the presentation of data that will be required for the FDA to eventually grant a license allowing the pharmaceutical company to market the drug, i.e., a Product License Application (PLA).

Most psychiatrists do not become familiar with new psychotropic drugs until they enter the Phase III stage. At this point, reports often appear in psychiatric journals of Phase III clinical trials, and the generic name for the drug becomes familiar to the practicing psychiatrist. For example, Serzone is the trade name for the generic antidepressant nefazodone. Nefazodone was relatively well known by psychiatrists through reports in the literature during Phase III trials prior to marketing in 1995, but the trade name Serzone became known only as a marketing commercial.

Phase III studies usually enroll 500–2,000 patients in order to evaluate better the effectiveness of the medication and potential side effects. Phase III subjects tend to vary more in their characteristics than those subjects who were included in the Phase II studies in order to obtain the broadest range of data on both efficacy and safety. Phase III studies which are ongoing in a community are sometimes perceived as a referral opportunity by psychiatrists who have been unsuccessful in treating certain patients. These patients may be most willing to become subjects, yet they frequently do not meet the inclusion and exclusion criteria for the study because of either comorbidity or lack of clarity regarding diagnosis.

Following completion of Phase III studies, the drug company makes a New Drug Application (NDA) to the FDA containing all relevant data. The NDA is tens of thousands of pages and contains all relevant information regarding the drug. The FDA and the pharmaceutical company then may negotiate issues, such as what is an acceptable approach to describing and marketing the drug. For example, a discussion may develop between a pharmaceutical company and the FDA regarding how the action of the drug can be described in advertising. There may have been little debate between Bristol-Myers Squibb (the maker of Serzone) and the FDA as to the actual mechanisms of the agent (the data were clear), but the wording of the product insert was discussed in great detail.

Once the drug is marketed, the drug company enters Phase IV, or postmarketing surveillance. Most pharmaceutical companies will enroll as many as 12,000 and perhaps as many as 30,000 patients in postmarketing studies to determine what side effects occur. The goal of phase IV is to document side effects that have a 95% chance of actually occurring at least once in every 10,000 patients. Physicians are asked to report, usually in narrative form, any side effect which occurred while the subject is taking the drug. (It is not necessary to know that the side effect is actually caused by the drug.) In addition, certain laboratory data may be requested. Pharmacists and physicians use automated databases (for example, a database from a health maintenance organization can be used) as sources for recording these side effects. These findings, in turn, are used to update the package insert accompanying the prescription drug.

Problem Set

Reynolds et al. (1992) explored the response to a combination of nortriptyline and interpersonal psychotherapy for acute and continuation treatment of elderly patients with recurrent major depression. Seventy-three older adults (61 of whom completed treatment) were prescribed nortriptyline in doses sufficient to produce a steady state of 80–120 ng/ml at bedtime. In addition, all subjects engaged in interpersonal psychotherapy during weekly 50-minute sessions administered by experienced psychotherapists trained in this form of therapy for 9 weeks, which was decreased to every other week and every 3 weeks during the 16 weeks of continuation therapy. During acute treatment, patients not responding to this combination therapy also received brief adjunctive pharmacotherapy with lithium and perphenazine. Forty-eight, or 79%, of the subjects entering this study achieved "full remission," that is, a Hamilton Depression Rating Scale (HDRS) score of 10 or lower over the 16 weeks of continuation therapy. Ten patients did not respond (their HDRS never dropped below 15) and three achieved only partial remission (HDRS ranging from 11 to 14). The authors concluded that the use of nortriptyline plus interpersonal therapy for 9 weeks of acute therapy and 16 weeks of continuation therapy appeared to be associated with a good response and relatively low attrition.

Questions

1. What is the design of this study?

2. The attrition from this study was relatively low, i.e., 16%, or 12 patients, were removed from the study during screening or acute therapy. Reasons for attrition were treatment refusal or noncompliance ($n = 8$), medical problems contraindicating further use of nortriptyline ($n = 3$), and spontaneous remission during the 2-week psychotropic-drug–free observation period before the start of acute therapy ($n = 1$). Two additional patients were lost during continuation. One died and one left the study against medical advice. Therefore 81% of the subjects completed at least 26 weeks of acute therapy. Would you expect this high a compliance rate in a double-blind placebo-control trial?

3. What exclusion criteria would you have institute for a study of the treatment of ambulatory depression in older adults with a combination of an antidepressant medication and psychotherapy?

4. What would be the next logical step for these investigators?

5. Would it be ethical to refuse treatment to an individual entering this study?

Answers

1. This is a open trial. Neither therapists nor patients were "blind" to the therapy which they received and there was no control group. Open trials are often used to determine if there is reason to proceed with a controlled trial, such as a double-blind placebo-control study.

In fact, these authors did follow the period of continuation therapy with a double-blind assignment to either placebo maintenance conditions or maintenance on nortriptyline. In this placebo-control double-blind phase of the study, 25% of those assigned to the placebo relapsed, whereas none of the patients assigned to nortriptyline continuation relapsed.

2. Probably not. First, all subjects were receiving a known therapy, and that therapy was accepted therapy for the treatment of depression in an ambulatory care setting. As the clinicians working with the subjects knew that the subjects were taking specific medication, they could discuss the potential side effects of the medications and therefore encourage subjects to continue on medications to "ride out" the side effects. This would not have been the case if the clinician evaluating the patient were blind to whether the treatment might in fact be a placebo.

3. First, as most clinical trials require that subjects be recruited from the community (and these heterogeneous subjects were recruited through media announcements), a specific diagnosis and severity of depressive symptoms should be assessed to determine if they meet criteria for the study. In this case, the Schedule for Affective Disorders and Schizophrenia (SADS) was used to diagnose major depression, and the Hamilton Depression Rating Scale was used to determine the severity of the depression. Subjects were required to meet criteria for a major depressive episode and to score at least 17 on the HDRS after 14 days without psychotropic drugs. To enter the trial, subjects were required to be off all psychotropic medications for at least 2 weeks (in order to avoid the impact of previous medications on the study).

In addition, severe medical illness as well as significant cognitive dysfunction would have been reasons for excluding patients from the study. For example, if an individual were suffering from severe cardiovascular disease which might, during the course of therapy, require adjustment or discontinuation of the antidepressant medication, such patients should be eliminated from the study initially. As a form of psychotherapy was used in the study, cognitive dysfunction might prevent a subject from responding to the treatment being tested. In fact, the frequency of comorbid physical and psychiatric disorders was relatively rare in this sample of patients.

Finally, these investigators were concerned that they not include individuals who were experiencing a chronic and nonremitting depression which, at least clinically, is known to be resistant to therapy. Therefore, they required that each patient be experiencing at least a second life-time episode of major depression and to have had an interepisode wellness interval of at least 2 months but no longer than 2.5 years.

4. The next step for these investigators is not entirely clear given the complexity of the initial open trial. One obvious approach would be to initiate a true double-blind placebo-control study of long-term use of nortriptyline. Beginning a double-blind placebo-control study (that is, a study of subjects with or without nortriptyline therapy) at the end of this open trial, however, does not answer the basic

question regarding the efficacy of the initial combined therapy compared to individual therapies (nortriptyline or interpersonal psychotherapy).

Performing a double-blind placebo-control trial of the combined therapies, however, could be difficult. For example, how will the subjects (not to mention the investigators) be blind to the psychotherapy? What control for the psychotherapy group could be used? One could have subjects meet with a clinician for a short period of time as frequently as subjects meet for interpersonal psychotherapy and compare the relative efficacy of the psychosocial interventions. These investigators, however, chose to compare the combination of therapy to the individual therapies alone.

5. It certainly would not be ethical to refuse treatment to an individual who is suffering from severe and potentially suicidal major depression. These individuals were ambulatory and less severely depressed. Therefore these investigators could consider the possibility of a placebo group (such as placing patients on a wait list for 10–12 weeks, yet following them at regular intervals carefully to determine the course of their depressive illness). Many less severe depressions improve without treatment. The use of placebos in studies such as this is controversial, however, given that antidepressant medications (as well as the cognitive-based psychotherapy such as interpersonal psychotherapy) have been demonstrated to be significantly superior to placebos in treating major depressive disorders.

REFERENCES

Reynolds C.F., Frank E., Parel J.M., Imber S.D., Cornes C., Morycx R.K., Mazumdar S., Miller M.D., Pollock B.G., Rifai A.H., Stack J.A., George C.J., Houch P.R., Kupfer D.J. 1992. Combined pharmacotherapy and psychotherapy in the acute and continuation treatment of elderly patients with recurrent major depression: a preliminary report. *American Journal of Psychiatry* 49: 1687–1692.

Roose S.P., Glassman A.H., Addia E., Woodring S. 1994. Comparative efficacy of selective serotonin reuptake inhibitors and tricyclics in the treatment of melancholia. *American Journal of Psychiatry* 151: 1785–1789.

III

ANALYSIS AND INTERPRETATION OF RESULTS

10

DIAGNOSTIC TESTS AND SCREENING INSTRUMENTS

OBJECTIVES

- To evaluate the accuracy of a diagnostic test
- To assess the correspondence between two imperfect tests
- To consider the appropriate use of tests for clinical decision-making, case-finding, and epidemiologic surveys

CASE EXAMPLE

In the dexamethasone suppression test (DST) the synthetic steroid dexamethasone is administered and serum cortisol is then measured at specified intervals over 24 hours. Elevated serum cortisol levels support a diagnosis of major depression with melancholia. To validate the DST as a laboratory test for endogenous or melancholic depression, Carroll and colleagues (1981) made standard psychiatric assessments of a sample of inpatients and outpatients ($n = 368$) from a clinical psychiatric research unit at the University of Michigan Medical Center. The assessment procedure included patient and family interviews of psychiatric and family histories, a structured diagnostic interview—the Schedule of Affective Disorders–Schizophrenia (SAD-S)—to assign a Research Diagnostic Criteria (RDC) diagnosis, and abstracts of the clinical record. A multidisciplinary consensus conference that reviewed these clinical data assigned the diagnosis of melancholic (endogenous) depression to 58% of all patients ($n = 215$). Patients with nonendogenous depression and other psychiatric disorders ($n = 153$) were assigned to the control group. A second control group of normal subjects with no psychiatric history ($n = 70$) was also enrolled. All subjects were given a dose of dexamethasone at 11:30 P.M. Blood cortisol levels were measured on the following day at 8:00 A.M., 4:00 P.M., and 11:00 P.M. for inpatients and at 4:00 P.M. only for outpatients and controls. Nonsuppression of blood cortisol levels was designated as ≥5 micrograms/deciliter (μg/dL) following administration of dexamethasone. Forty-three percent of the melancholic patients had cortisol levels ≥5 μg/dL, and 96% of the nonmelancholic patients had cortisol levels below 5 μg/dL. Of the subjects with cortisol levels ≥5 μg/dL, 94% had been diagnosed as melancholic by the clinical conference. Four percent of normal subjects had cortisol levels ≥5 μg/dL.

INTRODUCTION

Previous chapters presented a variety of study designs for estimating the relationship between an exposure and an outcome. If the measurement of either the exposure condition or the outcome condition is subject to systematic inaccuracies, however, the estimates of effect will be distorted. When undertaking clinical research, an investigator needs a method that can quantify the degree of inaccuracy in categorizing subjects with respect to their exposure level or outcome status—in other words, for estimating *misclassification bias*.

Clinical diagnoses are always subject to a probability estimate. *Staphylococcus aureus* or cervical cancer can be diagnosed with high probability because tests that serve as "gold standards" are available—i.e., the tests have demonstrated excellent validity and reliability. In contrast, differential diagnosis of psychiatric illness depends on the accumulation of a variety of test results derived from clinical interviews and observation, family history, and treatment response, which to varying degrees support a specific diagnosis but do not provide conclusive evidence. With the increasing medicalization of psychiatry, a proliferation of more technologically sophisticated diagnostic tests, including genetic, endocrinologic, and electrophysiologic measures, have become available for refining diagnostic probability. Unfortunately, there is a good deal of confusion about what such tests can and cannot do. In this chapter, the DST study by Carroll et al. is used to illustrate how a clinician can evaluate (1) the accuracy of a diagnostic test, (2) the utility of a test for refining a differential diagnosis, and (3) the suitability of a test for other purposes, such as case-finding or epidemiologic studies.

VALIDITY AND RELIABILITY OF DIAGNOSTIC TESTS AND INSTRUMENTS

A diagnostic test or instrument should first and foremost provide an accurate or valid assessment of the index disorder and do so reliably over time. The validity of a new diagnostic test depends on the degree to which it corresponds to the di-

agnostic *gold standard* (i.e., the best set of measures available to clinicians for diagnosing the index disorder). Even a highly accurate (valid) diagnostic test, however, is of little use if it cannot be reliably duplicated over time. In other words, a
reliable diagnostic test provides the same diagnosis for a given individual regardless of who administers it or when it is administered (except, of course, when a patient is in remission or has recovered, as discussed on pp. 45–47). This provides a
particular challenge to psychiatric diagnosticians who may be on the track of a relatively stable trait disorder or of a state disorder with a more unpredictable course.
A reliable diagnostic test minimizes what may be considerable biologic variability in psychiatric illness and is minimally affected by the variability of test instruments and test administrators (intra-observer and interobserver variability). For
example, a reliable diagnostic test of major depression minimizes the degree to
which variability of mood from one day to the next influences the assessment.
Table 10–1 summarizes the qualities of a good diagnostic test.

Carroll and colleagues were concerned about both the validity and the reliability of the DST. The scientific literature included widely varying reports of its effectiveness in differentiating melancholic depression from other subtypes of depression not characterized by melancholia. Moreover, variability in administration
of the DST (e.g., in the size of the loading dose of dexamethasone used, in the
timing of blood sampling, and in the criterion for how high a level of cortisol
release would be considered abnormal) limited the comparability of published
studies. Thus, the aims of their study were twofold: (1) to measure the probability that the DST would yield the same diagnostic results as the best available clinical gold standard for the diagnosis of melancholic subtype and (2) to standardize
the administration of the DST in such a way as to maximize the reliability of
the test.

Carroll et al. used a battery of clinical assessment procedures (histories, symptom, and severity scales) and informants (patient, family, and clinicians) to arrive
at an expert consensus on the "true diagnosis." The procedure, often called the
LEAD standard (Longitudinal, Expert, and Available Data) (Spitzer, 1983) is the
commonly accepted approach to evaluating the accuracy of both standardized diagnoses and laboratory tests in psychiatry. Nevertheless, the investigators were not
sanguine about this approach. Their skepticism was later reinforced by a 5-year
follow-up study that confirmed the diagnosis of unipolar major depressive disor-

TABLE 10–1. Qualities of a good diagnostic test

- Gives a positive result when the "true" disease status is positive
- Gives a negative result when the "true" disease status is negative
- Gives a positive (or negative) result when other tests give a positive (or negative) result
- Gives the same result over time (when the factor being studied is stable)
- Gives the same result when administered by multiple persons
- Increases confidence that a patient who tests positive has the disorder
- Increases confidence that a patient who tests negative does not have the disorder

der in fewer than 50% of "cases" diagnosed by such consensus conferences (Clayton et al., 1992).

Nevertheless, when assessing the accuracy of a new diagnostic test or instrument, the first task of the psychiatric investigator is to assemble the best array of previously available diagnostic instruments in order to identify correctly, within the designated sample, "true" cases and "true" noncases (controls), keeping in mind that there is still some degree of error at work in these instruments. Once subjects have been classified, the putative diagnostic test is then administered to them and they are categorized as "test positive" or "test negative." The total number of "positives" and "negatives" diagnosed and "positives" and "negatives" measured by the new test or instrument are used in a 2 × 2 table as row and column sums (Table 10–2) to assess the accuracy of the test.

Using the LEAD procedure, Carroll and his colleagues identified 215 patients (58%) with endogenous (melancholic) depression and 153 patients with nonendogenous depressions or other psychiatric diagnoses. The DST was administered to the same sample. Table 10–3 compares melancholia status as designated by the LEAD and the DST. Based on a serum cortisol level of ≥5 μg/dL for a positive test, 99 subjects (27%) were identified as having melancholic depression and the remainder (269 subjects) as nonmelancholic.

Sensitivity and Specificity

The validity of a diagnostic test is measured by its sensitivity and specificity. These properties of a test are based on the proportions of the sample who are true positives, true negatives, false positives, and false negatives, as displayed in each of

TABLE 10–2. Two-by-two table of true disease status by diagnostic test outcome

		True Disease		
		(+)	(−)	
Diagnostic	(+)	True Positive a	False Positive b	$a + b$
Test				
Outcome	(−)	False Negative c	True Negative d	$c + d$
		$a + c$	$b + d$	$a + b + c + d$

TABLE 10–3. Two-by-two table of melancholia status as designated by the LEAD (gold standard) and the dexamethasone suppression test (DST)

		LEAD		
		Melancholia	Nonmelancholic Psychiatric Disorders	
DST	(+)	True Positive (a) 93	False Positive (b) 6	99
	(−)	False Negative (c) 122	True Negative (d) 147	269
		215	153	368

Data from Carroll et al., 1981

the four cells of a 2×2 table. "True positives" (cell *a*) are *cases on both* the gold standard and on the diagnostic test. "True negatives" (cell *d*) are *noncases on both* the gold standard and on the diagnostic test. In a world of perfect tests, all subjects would fall on the "on-diagonal" (cell *a* and cell *d*). In the real world of clinical psychiatry, there are always subjects with discrepant results who fall on the "off-diagonal": "false positives" (cell *b*) who are *noncases by the gold standard but cases by the diagnostic test*, and "false negatives" (cell *c*) who are *cases by the gold standard but noncases by the diagnostic test*.

Sensitivity (*SN*) is the probability of testing positive if the "true" disease status is positive and is calculated as:

$$\text{Sensitivity } (SN) = a / (a + c)$$

or

$$\text{True positives} / (\text{true positives} + \text{false negatives})$$

The *false-negative rate* is the difference between "1.00" and the sensitivity (1.00 − *SN*) and measures the probability of testing negative if the "true" disease status is positive.

Specificity (*SP*) is the probability of testing negative if the "true" disease status is negative and is calculated as:

$$\text{Specificity } (SP) = d \, / \, (b + d)$$

or

True negatives / (false positives + true negatives)

The *false positive rate* is the difference between "1.00" and the specificity $(1 - SP)$ and measures the probability of testing positive if the "true" disease status is negative.

Depending on the purpose for which the test is used, the criterion for a positive result on a diagnostic test can be adjusted to increase the likelihood of including cases or of excluding noncases, but not both simultaneously. In other words, sensitivity can only be improved at the expense of specificity, and vice versa. One can readily see how a flexible cutoff point could achieve improved sensitivity by imagining how subjects would move across cells in a 2 × 2 table (see Table 10–2) under altered criteria. If a test is made less stringent such that more subjects count as "test positive" (more subjects move from cells c and d to cells a and b, respectively), then the probability of being classified "true positive" will rise as the value in cell a is augmented. The probability of being classified as "true negative" will simultaneously decrease because the value in the d cell is diminished.

Test results from true positives and true negatives will be distributed along the continuum of possible results and will overlap to some degree. One could hypothetically achieve perfect sensitivity such that all "true positives" were "test positives" (no false negatives) by using an extreme adjustment to the cutoff point which included 100% of the test scores from among those with the disorder (Figure 10–1). But the corresponding rise in false positive cases would delay the accurate diagnosis and effective treatment of patients with other disorders. Excessive false positives may also cause clinicians to discount results of a test that "cries wolf," i.e., causes many patients who do not actually have the disorder to test positive. On the other hand, perfect specificity protects those without the disorder from the distress and inconvenience of being wrongly diagnosed—but delays the diagnosis of those with the disorder whose test results were less extreme.

Carroll and colleagues found that, with a cutoff level ≥5 μg/dL, the DST had a sensitivity of .43 (i.e., the test identified 43% of patients who received a positive LEAD diagnosis of melancholic depression). The DST had a specificity of .96 (i.e., the test identified 96% of patients who received a negative LEAD diagnosis).

In the case example, five different cutoff levels for the DST were examined (Table 10–4). When the cutoff point was less stringent (≥3 μg/dL), the DST identified only a few more than half the melancholic patients identified by the consensus conference ($SN = .53$). At the same time it misdiagnosed 15% of nonmelancholic patients as melancholic ($SP = .85$). At the other end of the spectrum, the investigators were able to achieve perfect specificity by setting the cutoff level at

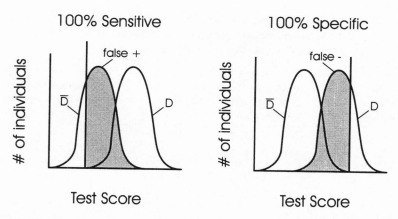

FIGURE 10–1. Improving sensitivity or specificity in a diagnostic or screening test for a disorder. Left: Perfect sensitivity can be achieved by shifting the cutoff value (vertical line) such that all individuals with the disorder (D) are captured, but many individuals without the disorder (D̄) are incorrectly diagnosed (indicated by shaded area). Right: Perfect specificity can be achieved by shifting the cutoff value for the same test such that it captures all persons who do not have the disorder (D̄); many individuals with the disorder (D) are incorrectly diagnosed (indicated by shaded area).

$\geq$10 μg/dL. At this level, none of the nonmelancholic patients exhibited abnormal cortisol levels. However, sensitivity was greatly reduced because only 15% of true melancholic patients exhibited cortisol levels as high as 10. The authors also examined the sensitivity and specificity of the DST under various conditions of administration, including the amount of steroid administered and the timing of serum cortisol testing, and ultimately recommended a $\geq$5 μg/dL cutoff point for a standardized administration procedure.

Predictive Value

Whereas sensitivity and specificity describe the accuracy of a test in a population, the diagnostic confidence or *predictive value* of a test estimates the probability that an individual case from the same population has been correctly diagnosed for the disorder by the test. The *positive predictive value* of a diagnostic test measures the degree to which a clinician may be confident that a positive test score signifies an increased probability that the patient has the disorder. It is calculated as the proportion of true positives among all subjects who test positive (see Table 10–1):

$$\text{Positive predictive value} = a / (a + b)$$

or

True positives / (true positives + false positives)

TABLE 10–4. Sensitivity and specificity of the Dexamethasone Suppression Test (DST) utilizing the 4:00 P.M. plasma cortisol concentration (μg/dL) among 215 patients with melancholia and 153 patients with other psychiatric disorders

PLASMA CORTISOL LEVEL (μg/dL) ≥	SENSITIVITY (PROBABILITY OF POSITIVE DST GIVEN TRUE MELANCHOLIA)	SPECIFICITY (PROBABILITY OF NEGATIVE DST GIVEN TRUE NONMELANCHOLIA)
3	53%	85%
4	48%	94%
5	43%	96%
6	39%	97%
10	15%	100%

Data from Carroll et al., 1981

The degree of confidence that negative results denote the absence of the disorder is called the *negative predictive value*, and is calculated as follows:

$$\text{Negative predictive value} = d / (c + d)$$

or

True negatives / (false negatives + true negatives)

Negative predictive value measures the confidence with which a clinician may rule out a diagnosis for a patient with a negative test result.

In the case example, of those identified by the DST with a cutoff of ≥5 μg/dL (Table 10–3), 94% were classified as melancholic by the LEAD (i.e., its positive predictive value was .94). At the same time, the researchers noted that of all subjects identified as nonmelancholic by the DST, only 55% were actually nonmelancholic on the LEAD rating (i.e., a negative predictive value of .55). Thus, patients for whom the estimated probability of melancholia is high (based on other test results) and whose cortisol levels exceed the DST cutoff value should be considered significantly more likely to have received an accurate diagnosis. Patients whose DST is normal do not have melancholia ruled out; rather, the estimated probability of melancholia is moderately diminished for them.

Predictive value, or diagnostic confidence, is influenced by the prevalence of the disorder in the population. A test with fixed sensitivity and specificity will have less predictive value when a disorder is rare in the sample tested because most positive results will be false, regardless of the specificity of the test. Diagnostic confidence in test results is greatest when used in populations where prevalence of the disorder is high, resulting in a high yield of positive cases. Thus, the transfer of a given test technology from a specialty clinical setting to a more diverse clinical setting can be treacherous.

For example, the diagnostic confidence associated with the DST in a mood-disorders clinic will be very different from its diagnostic confidence in a primary care setting where not only is the prevalence of melancholia much lower but (as noted by Carroll et al., 1981) diagnostic confusion about depressive subtypes is much higher. Consider a busy internal medicine practice where the prevalence of major depression among all the patients is hypothetically .06 (three times the population prevalence of .02), and 20% of these are melancholic. If an internist tried to identify—from all patients in the practice who complained of a persistent period of feeling blue—215 truly melancholic patients (the same number of patients with true melancholia as in the Carroll study), the proportion of true-positive DSTs would be smaller than in a tertiary care site with a higher prevalence of melancholia. Table 10–5 displays hypothetical cell and marginal frequencies for a large sample with prevalence of melancholia set to .012 (20% of .06), and sensitivity and specificity set at .43 and .96, respectively.

In this example, the positive predictive value of the DST would be approximately .12 and the negative predictive value over .99. Thus, the general internist

TABLE 10–5. Hypothetical 2×2 table of melancholia by LEAD (gold standard) and dexamethasone suppression test if prevalence were 1.2%

		LEAD		
		Melancholia	Nonmelancholia	
DST	(+)	93	708	801
	(−)	122	16,994	17,116
		215	17,702	17,917

could conclude with some justification that a patient who tested negative on the DST was most likely not melancholic. However, a positive screen would yield little diagnostic certainty that the patient was a "true melancholic" patient. Furthermore, such marginal certainty comes at a cost to patients and medical resources, multiplied many times for all the false positives.

Kappa

Where no gold standard is available for evaluating a new test (as is the case almost always in psychiatry), the ability of the new test to reproduce the results of another "imperfect" test may be measured using the *kappa coefficient* (Byrt et al., 1993), a measure of agreement (or reliability). Kappa is the coefficient of reproducibility appropriate for diagnostic tests with two levels: present and absent. Kappa has the advantage of taking into account the possibility that the two tests could agree by chance alone even if the true correspondence were nil. Kappa measures the distance between random 50% agreement and the actual agreement as a fraction of the distance between 50% agreement and 100% agreement. Thus, for:

Agreement =	Kappa	
50% (random chance)	0	
70%	.40	(i.e., 70% is 0.40 of the distance between 50% and 100%)
90%	.80	(i.e., 90% is 0.80 of the distance between 50% and 100%)
95%	.90	(i.e., 95% is 0.90 of the distance between 50% and 100%)
100% (perfect)	1.00	(i.e., 100% = 1.00 × the distance between 50% and 100%)

Generally, kappas of .40 may be considered acceptable, and .50–.65 would be considered good. The calculation of the kappa coefficient, based on probability theory, uses the cell and marginal frequencies, an example of which follows:

$$\text{Kappa} = \frac{\text{Observed agreement} - \text{chance-expected agreement}}{(1 - \text{chance-expected agreement})}$$

where observed agreement =

$$\frac{(a + d)}{(a + b + c + d)}$$

and Chance-expected agreement =

$$\frac{[(a + b) \times (a + c)] + [(c + d) \times (b + d)]}{(a + b + c + d)^2}$$

For example, the kappa coefficient for the data shown in Table 10–2 measures the chance-corrected agreement between the LEAD procedure and the DST. It is calculated as follows:

$$\text{Observed agreement} = (93 + 147) / 368 = .652174$$

$$\text{Chance-expected agreement} = \frac{(99 \times 215) + (269 \times 153)}{(368)^2} = .461085$$

$$\text{Kappa} = \frac{(.652174 - .461085)}{(1 - .461085)} = \frac{.191089}{.538915} = .354581 = .35$$

Thus, although the investigators observed a 65% agreement rate between the LEAD and the DST, they might have observed a 46% agreement rate by chance alone. After correcting for chance agreement, the DST reproduced the results of the LEAD approximately one-third of the time.

Kappa is designed for nominal classifications. When categories are ordinal (cf. Chapter 12), weighted kappas describe the closeness of agreement between ratings (Spitzer et al., 1967).

The kappa coefficient, as predictive value, is influenced by the prevalence of the disorder in the population being tested. Therefore, before accepting a given level of reproducibility between two tests in a study population on the basis of a kappa value derived from a different population, investigators should consider whether the disorder of interest was similarly distributed in their study population and in the population in which the kappa was quantified (Byrt et al., 1993).

SCREENING

Screening is usually defined as the application of a diagnostic test to "asymptomatic" persons for the purpose of classifying them with respect to the likelihood of having a particular disorder. In this sense of the term, screening has not commonly been undertaken for psychiatric disorders because observable symptoms have been the only bellwether of psychiatric pathology. Where psychiatric disorders are concerned, screening efforts have identified numerous persons who have symptoms but who are unknown to treatment providers. Psychiatric screening instruments, such as the Center for the Epidemiologic Studies–Depression (CES-D)

TABLE 10–6. Disorders favorable for screening

- Have serious consequences relative to the cost of screening
- Have high prevalence in the screened population
- Have improved prognosis with early detection
- Have a "good" screening test available

scale (Radloff, 1977) and the Beck Depression Inventory (Beck, 1967), are frequently used in primary care settings to advance a diagnosis of depression, especially given the low help-seeking behaviors associated with some psychiatric symptoms. Screening is sometimes undertaken in populations of individuals at particular risk of psychiatric complications (Table 10–6). This has perhaps been most successful when depressive symptom scales have been administered in selected demographic or life-cycle subgroups, such as postpartum females or medically ill elders. More general applications of psychiatric screening have occurred on days designated by community groups for newspaper surveys or special screening efforts in shopping malls. Instrumentation is usually a symptom checklist constructed with relatively high sensitivity, and potential cases are encouraged to seek follow-up testing.

Choosing the best screening test involves balancing the costs of false diagnoses vs. the costs of missing a true case. *Serial testing* (Figure 10–2) can be used to improve the specificity of a highly sensitive test because some false positives on the first test are likely to be converted to true negatives by the second test. For example, a relatively easy test to administer such as a PAP smear, which is extremely sensitive to cellular changes representing a very serious disease (cervical cancer) and which can be followed by a more specific test to rule out less serious problems, can afford to be more sensitive at the cost of specificity. However, sensitivity is sacrificed in any serial testing protocol because false negatives on the first test do not have a second chance to be diagnosed as true positives by the second test.

Parallel testing—in which all subjects testing positive on either of two different diagnostic tests are considered cases—improves sensitivity. For example, a research protocol may call for newly admitted psychiatric patients to be screened into a case group of depressed subjects either by scoring high on a symptom checklist such as the Center for Epidemiologic Studies–Depression scale (Radloff, 1977) or by receiving a clinical diagnosis of a depressive disorder. In this case of parallel testing, specificity is sacrificed because false positives may accumulate in the pool of cases from each of two diagnostic tests.

Screening programs for case-finding are evaluated by two criteria: feasibility and efficacy. Feasibility depends on the acceptability of screening instruments to the patients being tested. Inconvenient, uncomfortable, or expensive screening tests will be more often avoided or resisted by patients and volunteers. A screen-

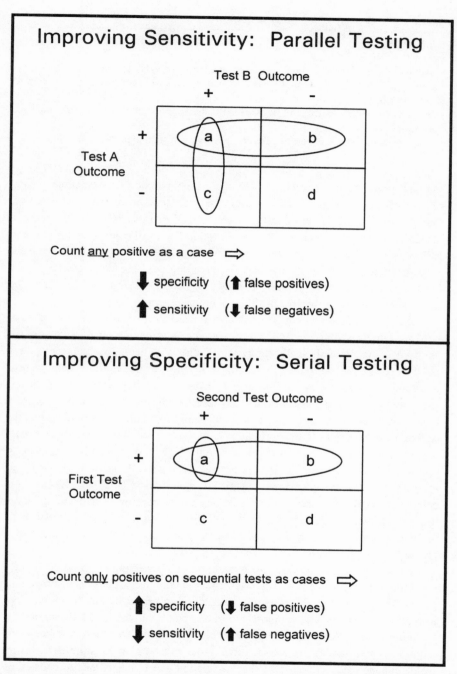

FIGURE 10–2. Sensitivity of a screening procedure can be improved by parallel testing (top) while specificity can be improved by serial testing (bottom).

TABLE 10–7. Qualities of a good screening test

- Inexpensive
- Easy to administer
- Minimally uncomfortable (both physically and emotionally) to patients
- Detects a disorder earlier than would occur if symptoms were severe enough to prompt help-seeking
- Balances the ability to detect most cases of the disorder with the ability to rule out noncases
- Not subject to variability across different testers or across time in the same tester

ing test should "do no harm," i.e., not cause undue anxiety among subjects who test positive and not give a false sense of security to subjects who test negative. Qualities of a good screening test are summarized in Table 10–7. Furthermore, a screening program is predicated on the availability of diagnosis, treatment, and follow-up for all screened persons. Feasibility, especially in today's health care environment, depends also on the cost of screening per case detected. Excessive cost–benefit ratios or low yield (even under the conditions of low cost) will not be acceptable in resource-limited health care environments.

The efficacy of a screening program is evaluated by comparing the outcomes of persons who were diagnosed by the screening test to the outcomes of persons diagnosed as a result of clinically emergent symptoms. Several questions may be applied to screening programs in psychiatric settings. (1) Does the screening program identify the psychiatric illness or subtype earlier than would be the case if the screen were not in place? (2) Do early stages of the disorder routinely progress to late-stage disorder, rather than being self-resolving? This is a critical issue, given that many "diagnoses" of depression or anxiety are self-resolving. (3) Does earlier treatment for the disorder improve prognosis, e.g., decrease the length of an episode, increase the remission time between episodes, decrease the severity of episodes, or prevent catastrophic sequelae of the disease? This issue, too, is critical in psychiatry, given that screening for depression in primary care among elders has been shown not to improve outcomes (Callahan et al., 1994). If the answers to these questions are affirmative, then screening tests may be an effective way to decrease the long-term burden of psychiatric illness.

Two sources of bias threaten the evaluation of a screening program. Volunteer (or self-selection) bias occurs when screening is voluntary. It has been shown that persons who volunteer for research and screening protocols are healthier, have lower mortality rates, and are more generally compliant with health regimens. On the other hand, volunteers may be more likely to be the "worried well" and (although asymptomatic) to have medical, family history, or lifestyle risk factors which enhance their propensity to seek a screening test. Schechter and colleagues (1994) found that only a small proportion of "normal" control subjects met Research Diagnostic Criteria for "never mentally ill." Because volunteers may be both better protected against and/or more at risk for poor health outcomes, estimating the direction and magnitude of self-selection bias is difficult.

A second source of bias stems from the episodic nature of many psychiatric disorders. An individual may be screened positive during an exacerbation of symptoms, only to screen negative upon subsequent diagnostic workups because the disorder is in remission and not because the individual was falsely diagnosed as positive at the initial screen. Even some biologic markers, such as nonsuppression of cortisol following dexamethasone administration and shortened REM (rapid eye movement) latency, are state phenomena (associated with melancholia) and will therefore be missing when the disorder is in remission. When screening for disorders without durable biological markers, it is important for screening measures to build in assessments of the course of symptomatology in individual patients over time.

EPIDEMIOLOGIC SURVEYS

The utility of psychiatric diagnostic tests is not limited to determining whether individual patients suffer from a disorder and to screening at-risk populations. Diagnostic tests may also be used in epidemiologic surveys and other descriptive studies (cf. Chapter 5). An example of such a survey is the development and use of the Diagnostic Interview Schedule (Regier et al., 1985) by investigators in the U.S. Epidemiologic Catchment Area (ECA) study (cf. Chapter 6). However, the reader should be alerted in the context of this discussion of testing that no diagnostic test has immutable properties of validity and reliability or is universally useful for differential diagnosis, case-finding, and population prevalence studies. For this reason, many debates have arisen over the "true" prevalence of specific psychiatric disorders in the general population. The choice of a test or series of tests should be based on a clearly articulated purpose and should have been previously evaluated for such a purpose. All such tests, whether interview or rating scales or laboratory tests, can and should be evaluated for validity and reliability as described above. Only then can clinical and research goals be optimally achieved.

Problem Set

Several research groups have suggested that parietal hypometabolism and hemispheric asymmetry precede a clinical presentation of the symptoms of Alzheimer's disease. Alzheimer's disease (AD) is the most common form of mental impairment in late life, with a prevalence as high as 0.47 among individuals 85 years and older. Gary Small and collaborators from California, New Mexico, North Carolina, and Massachusetts were searching for a test which could identify altered brain metabolism in cognitively asymptomatic individuals at risk of Alzheimer's disease by virtue of a family history of dementia and genotype (Small et al., 1995). Using APOE-4 status as

TABLE 10–8. Diagnosis of Alzheimer's disease by two PET scan tests (at stringent and less-stringent cutoff levels), in asymptomatic relatives of AD patients with (+) and without (−) APOE-4 allele, and in probable AD patients with dementia

PET SCAN DIAGNOSTIC TEST/ STRINGENCY OF CUTOFF CRITERIA	DIAGNOSIS AS AD CASE OR NONCASE	TEST RESULT	RELATIVES WITH APOE-4 (+)	(−)	PATIENTS WITH PROBABLE AD
Left parietal metabolism ratio					
Stringent cutoff	Case	<.85	7	6	6
Stringent cutoff	Noncase	≥.85	5	13	1
Less-stringent cutoff	Case	<.88	9	9	7
Less-stringent cutoff	Noncase	≥.88	3	10	0
Parietal asymmetry score					
Stringent cutoff	Case	>2.5	6	4	5
Stringent cutoff	Noncase	≤2.5	6	15	2
Less-stringent cutoff	Case	>1.8	8	7	7
Less-stringent cutoff	Noncase	≤1.8	4	12	0

Data from Small et al., 1995

their state-of-the art measure of "true disease," the investigators classified 31 asymptomatic relatives of probable AD patients according to their genotype, based on previous findings that the APOE-4 allele (the apolipoprotein E locus on chromosome 19) conveys significant risk of disease in a dose-response pattern. Twelve relatives of probable AD patients, all with APOE genotype 3/4, were classified as APOE-4(+), while 19 (17 with genotype 3/3 and two with 3/2) were classified as APOE-4(−). Seven demented patients with probable AD were also enrolled.

Subjects in all three groups received positron emission tomography (PET) scans. Left parietal metabolism ratios were <.85 (lower ratios signify decreased synaptic activity and greater probability of being a case) in seven APOE-4(+) relatives, six APOE-4(−) relatives, and six probable AD patients. A less stringent cutoff level of <.88 on the metabolism ratio would have included all seven probable AD patients as well as nine APOE-4(+) relatives and nine APOE-4(−) relatives (Table 10–8.)

Parietal asymmetry scores were >2.5 (higher scores signify greater probability of being affected) for six APOE-4(1) relatives, four APOE-4(−) relatives, and five probable AD patients. A less stringent cutoff level of >1.8 on the asymmetry score would have included all seven probable AD patients as well as eight APOE-4(1) relatives and seven APOE-4(2) relatives (Table 10–8).

Questions

1. Is there a gold standard for a diagnosis of Alzheimer's disease at the present time? What implications would such a standard have for diagnostic certainty in clinical psychiatric practice? What other criteria for diagnosis of AD are available to clinicians and acceptable to patients, and what degree of certainty do they convey?

2. In the two blank 2 × 2 tables provided (Table 10–9), plot the cell and mar-

TABLE 10–9. Blank 2×2 tables for questions 2(a) and 2(b)

a)

		APOE-4	
		(+)	(−)
Left Parietal	<.85		
Metabolism Ratio	≥.85		

b)

		APOE-4	
		(+)	(−)
Parietal Asymmetry	>2.5		
Score	≤2.5		

ginal frequencies for cases [APOE-4(+)] and controls [APOE-4(−)] among relatives of probable AD patients according to the results of each screening test reported by Small and colleagues:

(a) parietal metabolism ratios (cutoff<.85)

(b) asymmetry scores (cutoff <2.5)

Calculate the sensitivity, specificity, false-positive and false-negative rates, the kappa coefficient, and the positive and negative predictive values of each PET measure. Describe in words the interpretation of each measure of validity calculated above.

3. Of what utility to the study was the enrollment of symptomatic "probable AD" patients?

4. What are the pros and cons of making these screening tests for AD more sensitive (less stringent)? More specific (more stringent)? Would you recommend a screening test for AD which had perfect sensitivity? Why or why not?

Answers

1. A brain biopsy demonstrating the characteristic pattern of plaques and tangles coupled with clinical symptoms and signs of Alzheimer's disease prior to death would provide the best estimate of the probability of AD. Impractical in the extreme, a biopsy is not a suitable means for differentiating living demented patients who do and do not have AD. Psychiatrists typically diagnose AD based on patient- and informant-reported behavioral symptoms; standardized psychiatric and neurological evaluations using criteria such as those in *DSM-IV* (1994) and the NINCDS-ADRDA criteria (McKhann et al., 1984); and magnetic resonance imaging (MRI) scans to detect cerebral atrophy and to rule out other causes for cognitive symptoms. To date, all of these have been dependent on a patient's being well within the clinical disease phase of the illness and, even then, they are inconclusive (Galasko et al., 1994; Jobst et al., 1994; Johnson et al., 1994; Victoroff et al., 1995). Recent genetic work suggests that an abnormality at the apolipoprotein E locus on chromosome 19, particularly homozygotic pairs of APOE-4, raises the probability of future development of AD.

2(a). Using a cutoff level for hypometabolism ratio of <.85, the PET demonstrated a .58 probability of identifying individuals at high genotypic risk of developing AD and a .68 probability among individuals at low genotypic risk of developing AD. The PET demonstrated a .42 probability of erroneously classifying those at high genotypic risk as low risk by virtue of a high metabolic ratio and a .32 probability of erroneously classifying those at low genotypic risk as high risk

2(a). **TABLE 10–10.** Two-by-two table of APOE-4 genotype status by magnitude (low vs. high) of left parietal metabolism ratio among relatives of symptomatic AD patients

		APOE-4		
		(+)	(−)	
Left Parietal	<.85	7	6	13
Metabolism Ratio	≥.85	5	13	18
		12	19	31

SN = .58   False-Negative Rate = .42
SP = .68   False-Positive Rate = .32
Kappa coefficient = .26
Positive Predictive Value = .54
Negative Predictive Value = .72

Data from Small et al., 1995

by virtue of their low metabolic ratio. The chance-corrected agreement between the two tests was .26. The likelihood was .54 that the parietal metabolism ratio would correctly identify AD relatives at high genotypic risk and .72 that it would correctly identify AD relatives at low genotypic risk.

2(b). Using a cutoff level for parietal asymmetry of >2.5, the PET demonstrated a .50 probability of identifying individuals at high genotypic risk of developing AD and a .79 probability among individuals at low genotypic risk of developing AD. The PET demonstrated a .50 probability of erroneously classifying those at high genotypic risk as low risk because the parietal asymmetry score was below the cutoff and a .21 probability of erroneously classifying those at low genotypic risk as high risk by their high parietal asymmetry scores. The chance-corrected agreement between the two tests was .30. The likelihood was .60 that the parietal asymmetry score would correctly identify AD relatives at high genotypic risk and .71 that it would correctly identify of AD relatives at low genotypic risk.

2(b). **TABLE 10–11.** Two-by-two table of APOE-4 genotype status by magnitude (high vs. low) of parietal asymmetry among relatives of symptomatic AD patients

		APOE-4		
		(+)	(−)	
Parietal Asymmetry Score	>2.5	6	4	10
	≤2.5	6	15	21
		12	19	31

SN = .50   False-Negative Rate = .50
SP = .79   False-Positive Rate = .21
Kappa coefficient = .30
Positive Predictive Value = .60
Negative Predictive Value = .71

Data from Small et al., 1995

3. The symptomatic patients provide an alternative "true disease" group which can assist in evaluating cutoff levels which were perfectly sensitive, i.e., captured all the probable AD cases.

4. Improved or perfect sensitivity would increase the likelihood of identifying all persons at risk of developing AD, but unless proven curative or significant palliative treatments emerge, the clinical worth of increased lead time is debatable. Furthermore, the anguish associated with the corresponding increase in false pos-

itives would seem untenable. On the other hand, a more specific test would give false confidence to an increasing proportion of relatives of AD patients who might otherwise make financial or treatment arrangements based on a higher likelihood of developing the disease. In a research setting, however, increased sensitivity is of urgent importance for the selection of at-risk subjects for preventive intervention trials.

REFERENCES

Beck A.T. 1967. *Depression: Causes and Treatment*. Philadelphia: University of Pennsylvania Press.

Byrt T., Bishop J., Carlin J.B. 1993. Bias, prevalence, and kappa. *Journal of Clinical Epidemiology* 46: 423–429.

Callahan C.M., Hendrie H.C., Dittus R.S., Brater D.C., Hui S.L., Tierney W.M. 1994. Improving treatment of late life depression in primary care: a randomized clinical trial. *Journal of the American Geriatrics Society* 42: 839–846.

Carroll B.J., Feinberg M., Greden J.F., Tarika J., Albala A.A., Haskett R.F., James N.M., Kronfol Z., Lohr N., Steiner M., de Vigne J.P., Young E. 1981. A specific laboratory test for the diagnosis of melancholia: Standardization, validation, and clinical utility. *Archives of General Psychiatry* 38: 15–22.

Clayton P.J., Guze S.B., Cloninger C.R., Martin R. L. 1992. Unipolar depression: diagnostic inconsistency and its implications. *Journal of Affective Disorders* 26: 111–116.

DSM-IV. 1994. *Diagnostic and Statistical Manual of Mental Disorders: DSM-IV*, 4th ed. Washington, DC: American Psychiatric Association.

Galasko D., Hansen L.A., Katzman R., Wiederholt W., Masliah E., Terry R., Hill L.R., Lessin P., Thal L.J. 1994. Clinical-neuropathological correlations in Alzheimer's disease and related dementias. *Archives of Neurology* 51: 888–895.

Jobst K.A., Hindley N.J., King E., Smith A.D. 1994. The diagnosis of Alzheimer's disease: a question of image? *Journal of Clinical Psychiatry* 55(*Suppl.*): 22–31.

Johnson J., Sims R., Gottlieb G. 1994. Differential diagnosis of dementia, delirium, and depression. Implications for drug therapy. *Drugs and Aging* 5: 431–445.

McKhann G., Drachman D., Folstein M., Katzman R., Price D., Stadlan E.M. 1984. Clinical diagnosis of Alzheimer's disease: report of the NINCDS-ADRDA Work Group under the auspices of Department of Health and Human Services Task Force on Alzheimer's Disease. *Neurology* 34: 939–944.

Radloff L.S. 1977. The CES-D Scale: a self-report depression scale for research in the general population. *Applied Psychological Measures* 1: 385–401.

Regier D.A., Myers J.K., Kramer M., Robins L.N., Blazer D.G., Hough R.L., Eaton W.W., Locke B.Z. 1985. Historical context, major objectives, and study design. In *Epidemiologic Field Methods in Psychiatry: The NIMH Epidemiologic Catchment Area Program* (eds. Eaton W.W., Kessler L. G.), pp. 3–19. Orlando, FL: Academic Press.

Schechter D., Strasser T.J., Santangelo C., Kim E., Endicott, J. 1994. "Normal" control subjects are hard to find: a model for centralized recruitment. *Psychiatry Research* 53: 301–311.

Small G.W., Mazziotta J.C., Collins M.T., Baxter L.R., Phelps M.E., Mandelkern M.A., Kaplan A., La Rue A., Adamson C.F., Chang L., Guze B.H., Corder E.H., Saunders

A.M., Haines J.L., Pericak-Vance M.A., Roses A.D. 1995. Apolipoprotein E type 4 allele and cerebral glucose metabolism in relatives at risk for familial Alzheimer Disease. *Journal of the American Medical Association* 273: 942–947.

Spitzer R.L. 1983. Psychiatric diagnosis: are clinicians still necessary? *Comprehensive Psychiatry* 24: 399–411.

Spitzer R.L., Cohen J., Fleiss J.L., Endicott J. 1967. Quantification of agreement in psychiatric diagnosis. *Archives of General Psychiatry* 17: 83–87.

Victoroff J., Mack W.J., Lyness S.A., Chui H.C. 1995. Multicenter clinicopathological correlation in dementia. *American Journal of Psychiatry* 152: 1476–1484.

11

Population Genetics Studies

OBJECTIVES

- To describe the methodology and methodological issues associated with population genetic studies, including determination of zygosity, case identification, and stability of diagnosis.
- To describe the relationship between population genetics and molecular genetics through linkage studies.
- To explain the concept of heritability, including multifactorial inheritance and penetrance, and the quantitative methods for determining heritability.
- To describe the design of twin studies and twin/adoption studies.

CASE EXAMPLE

Fifteen years ago Egeland and Hostetter (1983) reported that bipolar mood disorder (manic-depressive illness) exhibited significant heritability among the Amish. In many ways, the Amish are an ideal population in which to study the heritability of psychiatric disorders. They are relatively isolated, have large families, and are descended from approximately 50 couples who arrived in Pennsylvania from Germany about 250 years ago. In addition, alcohol and drug abuse among the Amish is rare. In a pedigree study Egeland and Hostetter found a pattern of inheritance of manic-depressive illness that suggested the illness is inherited via a dominant gene with incomplete penetrance (35–55% of those who inherit the gene eventually develop manic-depressive illness). In a later study Egeland and colleagues (1989) performed a linkage study in which they determined that some cases of manic depression are caused by a dominant gene on the tip of the short arm of chromosome 11. Though this study has been widely criticized, it was one of the first instances in which molecular genetic techniques were applied to a population genetic study of a psychiatric disorder.

INTRODUCTION

The study designs described so far in this book are used most often to identify risk factors for psychiatric disorders without distinguishing between factors that are innate or acquired. For example, gender is an innate characteristic whereas the exposure to a stressful event, such as the death of a parent, is acquired. Investigators are increasingly aware of the necessity of separating risk factors that are innate (and therefore inherited) from those that are acquired from the physical and psychosocial environment. Inherited risk factors suggest a very different approach to prevention and treatment compared to environmental risk factors.

Special methods have been developed to determine the extent to which hereditary factors increase the risk for developing a psychiatric disorder compared to environmental factors. The details of these methodologies are complex and beyond the scope of this book. Nevertheless, this chapter should give the reader a basis for understanding the many studies published in psychiatric journals that use the methods of population genetics as distinguished from the methods of molecular genetics.

Population genetics focuses on the contribution of genetic and environmental factors to observable behaviors among persons in populations (phenotypes). The usual subjects for population genetic studies derive from pedigree and twin samples. Pedigrees are family trees, as illustrated in Figure 11–1. Twin samples are usually drawn from twin registries, such as the registries available in Scandinavian countries (see below). Population genetics complements molecular genetics by describing the frequency and distribution of phenotypes in human populations and exploring factors that change these frequencies and distributions.

Molecular-genetic techniques are directed at locating the gene or combination of genes that produce those proteins responsible for the function of an organism. The techniques used in molecular genetics include recombinant DNA and genetic probes to map the genome and identify the gene or genes responsible for an observable behavior, such as a thought disorder.

The overlap of molecular genetics with population genetics occurs through linkage analysis. Linkage analysis is a statistical procedure applied to a family (a pedigree) in which a particular disease or abnormality is distributed. The analysis is

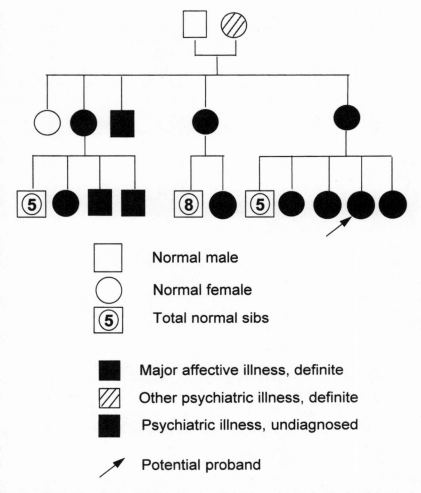

FIGURE 11–1. Inhertiance of major affective illness in an Amish family (partial reproduction of pedigree described by Egeland and Hostetter, 1983).

used to determine whether the genetic locus for a disease or behavioral expression is near, and therefore "cosegregates" with, a genetic marker on a particular chromosome. A genetic marker is a portion of the chromosome that has been located previously and therefore can be easily identified by molecular genetic techniques. The gene for Huntington's disease was identified on chromosome 4 by following the distribution of Huntington's disease through multiple generations in large family pedigrees via a known genetic marker on the chromosome closely linked to the Huntington gene. It had previously been established that Huntington's disease is caused by a single genetic abnormality. As Huntington's disease and the genetic marker are inherited together, i.e., they cosegregate, it can be assumed that the genetic abnormality causing the disease and the genetic marker are located near one another on the same chromosome. Molecular genetic techniques were then used to identify the previously unknown abnormal gene that causes Huntington's disease. Thus, population-genetic studies are critical to the molecular genetic exploration of human disease.

The modern history of population genetics began with Gregor Mendel during the middle of the 19th century. By studying his breeding experiments using different varieties of pea plants, most persons learned in high school or college about "Mendelian" genetic concepts such as autosomal dominant, autosomal recessive, and the two laws of heritability. The first law, the law of segregation, states that there are two "elements" or alleles of heredity for each observed characteristic and these alleles separate or segregate during the process of inheritance. In Figure 11–2 (a), the alleles for a particular gene are A_1 and A_2. The second law, the law of independent assortment, states that the inheritance of one trait does not influence the inheritance of another trait. In Figure 11–2 (b), the inheritance of one of the "A" alleles (A_1 or A_2) is independent of the inheritance of the "B" alleles (B_1 or B_2). (When they are not independent, they are linked.)

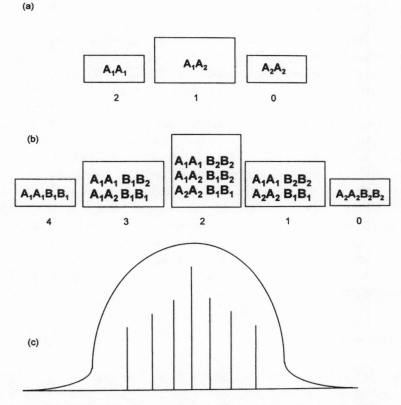

FIGURE 11–2. The change in distribution of traits, such as symptoms of depression, with increasing numbers of genes contributing to the trait. (Adapted from Plomin et al., 1990.)

Other concepts relevant to population genetics were developed around the same time Mendel worked with pea plants. For example, Charles Darwin introduced the concept of environmental modification, i.e., the spontaneous change of inherited characteristics and the natural selection for the fittest over time. A mutation in a gene which leads to a change in inherited characteristics, such as a change in skin color, may provide an advantage to an animal in a particular ecological niche, and therefore animals with that skin color would gradually become more prevalent and dominate other animals which did not experience the mutation. Frances Galton introduced the use of twins to assess the relative contribution of nature, i.e., inheritance, and the role of nurture, i.e., the environment, to the characteristics of children. During the first decade of this century, Hardy and Weinberg quantified an assumption regarding mating behavior. The Hardy-Weinberg law states that genotypic and allelic frequencies are stable from one generation to another. This equilibrium depends on random mating. Selective or assortative mating (as might occur among a few Scandinavian families moving to Minnesota), genetic drift (as when schizophrenics perhaps move down the socioeconomic ladder over time and intermarry), mutation, migration, and other selection factors undermine this equilibrium.

An example of the Hardy-Weinberg law is the frequency of cystic fibrosis in the Caucasian population of the United States, which is approximately one in 2,500 births. Cystic fibrosis is inherited as an autosomal recessive disorder. Therefore, the frequency of carriers of the single abnormal allele is one in 25. The risk of two carriers having a child with cystic fibrosis is one in four, and the risk for a sibling of someone with cystic fibrosis having a child with cystic fibrosis is one in 150. If random mating occurs, these figures do not change through time. The Amish studied by Egeland et al. do not practice random mating. They are an ultraconservative Protestant religious sect and tend to intermarry within their community (not within individual families, however). Though the relative isolation of these individuals makes it easier to identify cases through multiple generations and study the genetic transmission of psychiatric disorder, the nonrandom mating may mean that the results cannot be generalized to the population at large. In other words, one may not be able to apply the Hardy-Weinberg law of equilibrium to the Amish.

We will now discuss the specific types of methods of population-genetic studies, such as pedigree studies, twin studies and adoption studies, and the use of linkage analysis in such studies. The principles discussed above apply to all of the methods described.

PEDIGREE STUDIES

The Egeland and Hostetter study (1983) is an excellent example of a pedigree study that explored the Mendelian heritability of a psychiatric disorder. This study described the distribution of psychiatric disorders in a multigenerational family that included multiple members who experienced disorders, permitting the investigator to study the heritability of the disorder from one generation to another (or the lack thereof). A partial example of one of these pedigrees is presented in Figure 11–1. As can be seen, many persons with psychiatric disorders were found across multiple generations in this Amish family; the majority suffered from major affective illness (*major mood disorder* in our current nomenclature). Though Egeland and colleagues began by studying entire families, most pedigree studies begin with a proband, that is, a person in the family diagnosed with the disease of interest. Then the investigator attempts to study other family members.

The Egeland pedigree of the Amish family shows that major affective disorder is inherited as an autosomal dominant trait. If the genetic abnormality is "fully penetrant," a person will experience the disorder if she/he has one abnormal allele. A fully penetrant disorder is one that inevitably appears if the genetic abnormality is present. Most psychiatric disorders associated with a genetic abnormality are not fully penetrant, however, and this renders pedigree study less than ideal as demonstrated by the Egeland study. As demonstrated in Figure 11–1, autosomal dominant disorders are found in every generation. Approximately equal numbers of men and women received the diagnosis in the family pedigree exhibited. With fully penetrant abnormalities, if one parent carries the gene (and experiences the illness), one-half of the children will carry the gene and experience the illness. In the pedigree shown, fewer than one-half of offspring experience the disorder. This suggests partial penetrance for affective disorder. It should be recognized, however, that this pedigree is confined to one family where major affective disorder is frequent and is not representative of all the Amish families located in Lancaster County, Pennsylvania (where this study took place). In fact, the overall frequency of affective disorder in this community is perhaps lower than for society at large: Less than 1% of the more than 8,000 Amish residents of Lancaster County received a confirmed diagnosis of bipolar or unipolar affective disorder.

If a heritable illness is studied in an entire population, such as among the Amish of Lancaster County, the illness will be frequent in certain families (and in this case transmitted as an autosomal dominant in the families), whereas in other families it is distributed sporadically and infrequently (and is therefore of questionable heritable predisposition). The distribution of most cases of major affective disorder are sporadic. Even so, pedigree studies can be valuable in determining the mode of inheritance among families in which the disease is heritable. When pedigree studies are coupled with molecular-genetic studies through linkage studies, a gene or the genes responsible for the disorder in those families may be identified.

In autosomal recessive inheritance, if the disease is rare (as are most psychiatric disorders), parents and relatives of the proband (or of an affected individual) will usually not experience the disorder. However, if one parent carries the gene, then one-half of the children will carry the gene. If both parents carry the gene (but do not experience the disorder), one-fourth of the children will experience the disorder, one-half of the children will carry the gene but not experience the disorder, and one-fourth will not carry the gene. In x-linked dominant inheritance, mothers transmit the disorder to children in one-half of the cases, and fathers transmit the disorder to their daughters. In sex-linked recessive cases, mothers who are carriers of the gene but who do not experience the disorder transmit the gene to one-half of their daughters and the disorder to one-half of their sons. The daughters with only one abnormal gene do not experience the disorder, but the sons with the abnormal gene do experience the disorder.

Among the psychiatric disorders, few have emerged which follow a strictly Mendelian inheritance. As described above, bipolar disorder is thought to be transmitted as an autosomal-dominant gene in some families, but this is debated. Other investigators have suggested that bipolar disorder is an x-linked, dominant condition.

In a pedigree study, how does one determine exactly what a gene expresses? Investigators have access only to the "phenotype," i.e., the observable features of the person with or without the disorder. The phenotype results from the interaction between the genotype and the environment. Therefore, one must not assume that he or she can directly observe the expression of a gene, or even the combination of a series of genes, because investigators almost always observe the contribution of heredity through many layers of environmental influence. Even when they observe a person experiencing a disorder with a sizable hereditary contribution, such as schizophrenia, the environmental influence renders parcelling out the hereditary influence difficult. No two schizophrenic subjects behave exactly the same way. Even among identical twins who both develop schizophrenia, the age of onset will vary as well as the symptoms.

Other methodological issues that must be considered when performing and reviewing pedigree studies are not complicated. To determine whether a condition is inherited as a dominant, recessive, or x-linked trait and demonstrates complete penetrance, a visual review of the pedigree will usually provide the answer, as in Figure 11–1. In cases where such a review does not provide the answer, statistical adjustments can be made to take into account factors which mask complete penetrance. For example, a pedigree study of Alzheimer's disease may suggest the disease is inherited as autosomal dominant. However, because the onset of the condition may not occur until well into the eighth decade, early death of persons who carry the gene and therefore would develop the disorder if they lived long enough masks the inheritance pattern in the pedigree study. The methods for performing these statistical adjustments are beyond the scope of this book. In the Egeland and Hostetter article, the authors only reported the presence of the diagnoses among the Amish pedigrees which they studied without statistical analysis and therefore did not statistically adjust for incomplete penetrance. They reproduced examples of the pedigrees, as demonstrated in Figure 11–1.

Perhaps the most difficult methodological task in a pedigree study is locating family members across multiple generations and encouraging them to participate in the study. Given the mobility of our current society, coupled with the relative unwillingness of persons to participate in survey research, most geneticists who work with families have learned to "cultivate" these families. As noted above, pedigree studies usually begin in a clinic when a clinician makes a diagnosis, such as bipolar disorder, and discovers, by taking a family history, that many persons in the family suffer from a similar disorder. When such a family is identified, the population geneticist will work with the identified patient (the proband) to gain access to and cooperation from family members. Egeland and her colleagues worked for years to gain the confidence and cooperation of the Amish for their pedigree studies. Honesty, concern, protection of confidentiality, as well as an appeal to altruism facilitate participation.

Accurate case identification is the most critical requirement for a pedigree study after the investigator is assured that adequate family members have been identified for study. Issues associated with case identification do not vary from those which have been discussed elsewhere in this book (see Chapters 6, 10). For a study of heredity, however, the stability of the diagnosis over time is especially important. For example, if an episode of major depression is the first episode in a series of episodes which will eventually include both manic and depressive episodes, the diagnosis of bipolar disorder will only become manifest through time and only then will the individual be accurately classified for the genetic study. Therefore, working with families over long periods of time is essential to pedigree studies.

Establishing accurate diagnoses of family members not directly available for study presents a different challenge to the investigator. Medical records are frequently not available and, if available, may not be useful. Therefore, questionnaires have been developed and validated which can be administered to family members who know other family members not available for direct study. In the Egeland study, as seen in Figure 11–1, some persons not contacted could be accurately identified as experiencing a major affective disorder, whereas others could only be identified as experiencing some variety of psychiatric disorder.

LINKAGE STUDIES

The bridge between pedigree studies and molecular genetics is the linkage study. (Moldin et al., 1995) Linkage analysis, briefly described above, is a powerful method for identifying a locus on the genome associated with a disorder. The method employed in linkage analysis derives directly from the method of a typical pedigree study. A family is selected in which multiple members experience the psychiatric disorder. Perhaps the family is identified initially through a proband or perhaps a multigenerational family is known to an investigator through a community study, such as the study performed by Egeland and colleagues among the

Amish. Regardless, the methods for case identification across generations proceed as with any pedigree study.

A hypothesis is generated regarding the location of the gene which underlies the heritability of the disorder. For example, in a second study by Egeland and colleagues, they hypothesized that a dominant gene for bipolar disorder was located on chromosome 11 (Egland et al., 1987). The Egeland group, in association with investigators from the Massachusetts Institute of Technology, had been performing recombinant DNA studies on chromosome 11. The investigators hypothesized that the gene responsible for bipolar disorder was located near a portion of chromosome 11 which they had cloned, and therefore this portion of the chromosome served as a genetic marker for the location of the gene for bipolar disorder.

The statistical procedure used to determine whether there is linkage, i.e., whether the marker is near the hypothesized gene, produces an LOD (logarithm of the odds) score. If there is no linkage, the probability of recombination is 50%: The genetic abnormality segregates independently from the genetic marker. The usual convention is that an odds ratio of 1,000:1 in favor of linkage demonstrates linkage, and an odds ratio of 100:1 against linkage is evidence enough to reject linkage. (The reader should not confuse the discussion of odds ratio here and the discussion of odds ratio in Chapter 3). When geneticists use the logarithm to the base 10 of the odds ratio, i.e., the LOD score, a LOD score of 3 signifies linkage and a score of -2 LOD indicates nonlinkage. LOD scores can be summed across multiple pedigrees. In the Egeland et al. study, the LOD score calculated across multiple pedigrees was 4.08.

Despite the excitement generated by the initial linkage studies published by Egeland and her colleagues, these results have not been replicated, and further analyses of these pedigrees (with new diagnoses added and additional DNA typing for the genetic marker performed) lowered the LOD score below 3. Though linkage studies are ongoing in psychiatry, no major findings have emerged which are uniformly accepted by psychiatrists and which link a common psychiatric disorder to a single dominant or recessive gene.

TWIN STUDIES

The most powerful method for studying the relative contribution of heredity and environmental factors is through twin studies. Twin studies usually are performed using existing twin registries. A listing of representative twin registries which have been used in population genetic studies of psychopathology is provided in Table 11–1.

These studies depend upon distinguishing monozygotic (identical) twins from dizygotic (fraternal) twins. Monozygotic twins result from one zygote's division

TABLE 11–1. Examples of twin registries used as data sources for psychiatric epidemiology

National twin registries:
a) Population-based:
  Denmark: Danish Twin Register (Bertelsen et al., 1977)
  Finland: Finnish Twin Cohort (Kaprio, 1994)
  Norway: Norwegian twin registry (Tambs et al., 1995)
  Sweden: Swedish Twin Registry (Allgulander et al., 1991)
       Swedish Psychiatric Twin Registry (Roy et al., 1995)
  U. S.: National Academy of Sciences/National Research Council Twin Registry:
      White male twin pairs who served in military, born 1917–1927 (Page, 1995)
      Vietnam Era Twin Registry: male twin pairs who served in U.S. military
        between 1965 and 1975 (Tsuang et al., 1996)
b) Voluntary:
  Australia: Australian National Health and Medical Research Council Twin Register
      (Kendler et al., 1986)

Regional Twin Registries:
  U. K. (England): Maudsley Hospital Twin Register, London (McGuffin et al., 1996)
  U. S.: Minnesota Twin Family Registry (Lykken et al., 1990)
      Virginia Twin Registry (Kendler et al., 1995)

into two embryos. Dizygotic twins result from simultaneous fertilization of two ova by two sperm. Monozygotic twins have the same genetic makeup, and their physical appearance is usually very similar. Dizygotic twins appear no more alike than siblings. One means of determining zygosity, other than observation, is to ask the twins if they are so much alike that they would describe themselves as "two peas in a pod," which usually produces a 90+% accuracy in distinguishing monozygotic from dizygotic twins. Investigators now have the ability to genotype individuals to determine zygosity, i.e., to fingerprint individuals using DNA by means of a blood sample from which a pair of twins are compared for genetic markers. Twin studies can best be understood, however, within the context of adoption studies.

Twin studies, especially twin adoption studies, are valuable for determining the relative contributor of genetic and environmental factors because both contribute to psychopathology. In contrast, usual clinical studies, even studies that employ biological markers, cannot establish the relative contribution of these factors. (See section on Adoption Studies below for a description of methodological assumptions necessary for quantitative statistical calculations.) Yet twin adoption studies are more rare than traditional twin studies because they require twins to have been adopted at birth and thereafter to have been reared apart. Adoption studies which are not limited to twins and which are used to determine whether etiology contains a significant hereditary component are described below.

ADOPTION STUDIES

The Scandinavian countries have been the primary source of data for adoption studies. There is a reason for this. Today's prosperous Scandinavia was impoverished before and during World War I. Many families could not afford to rear their twin children and therefore offered one or both children for adoption in the hope of ensuring them a better life. The Scandinavians also kept meticulous records of adoption. This combination of unfortunate need and meticulous care provided an excellent population laboratory within which to disentangle the genetic and the environmental.

The basic design of the adoption study is presented in Figure 11–3. A child adopted from birth has both hereditary and environmental contributors to his/her phenotype. It is assumed that the biological parents (P_b) contribute only their genotypes to the phenotype (P) of the adopted offspring (Po). The adoptive parents (Pa) contribute only the environmental elements (e). There are three variations of this design. In the first variation, biological parents of adoptive children are identified as either suffering from a psychiatric disorder or as being without psychiatric illness. Then the frequency of illness in the adopted offspring is compared to the frequency in the biological offspring. Genetic contribution to the illness is indicated if the frequency of illness among adopted children of biological parents with the psychiatric disorder is greater than the frequency among adopted children of biological parents without the psychiatric disorder. A second design begins with the

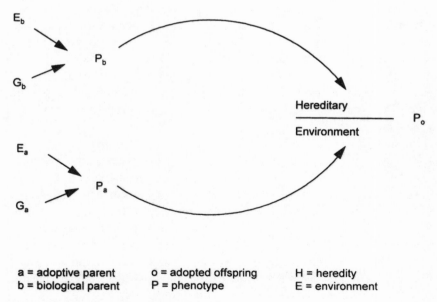

a = adoptive parent   o = adopted offspring   H = heredity
b = biological parent   P = phenotype   E = environment

FIGURE 11-3. Basic design of adoption studies.

identification of adopted children who have experienced a psychiatric disorder. In this design, genetic factors are assumed to contribute to the disorder if the frequency of the illness in the biological parents of the children is greater than in the adoptive parents. The third design is a "cross-fostering" approach, an approach which compares the overall frequency of illness in two groups of adoptees, one group having ill biological parents and raised by well adoptive parents, whereas the other group have well biological parents and is raised by ill adoptive parents. This design can be extended to include an analysis of relatives other than parents.

As illustrated in Figure 11–3, environmental and hereditary influences both contribute to the psychopathology (or lack of psychopathology) in the parent of the adopted offspring. The adopted offspring, however, is only affected by environmental influences from the adoptive parent and genetic influences of the biological parent.

There are many potential flaws in the design of adoptive studies. First, adoptive studies do not take into account the shared environment of twins prior to birth. Second, these studies do not take into account shared parent–child interaction from the time of birth to the separation of siblings by adoption (which may be months to years following birth). In many adoptive studies, it is not clear exactly when the parent was separated from the child, though the Scandinavian countries generally are able to identify time of adoption compared to time of birth.

Perhaps the best-known early example of an adoption study was performed by Kety and colleagues in Denmark (Kety et al., 1976). These investigators began with 507 individuals who had been admitted to a psychiatric facility. Thirty-three were classified as cases of schizophrenia who had been adopted from birth (the probands). Then Denmark public records were searched for names of the biological parents, siblings, and other relatives as well as the adoptive families. Nearly all of the biological parents and adoptive parents were identified. Approximately 90% of the relatives were actually interviewed (where warranted) and a psychiatric diagnosis was assigned by consensus. The results of the study are presented in Table 11–2.

As can be seen, there is approximately a fourfold increase in the frequency of schizophrenia among biological relatives compared to adoptive relatives. These data, therefore, suggest that there is an hereditary contribution to schizophrenic

TABLE 11–2. Example of an adoption study

	NONSCHIZOPHRENIC ADOPTEES	SCHIZOPHRENIC ADOPTEES
First degree biological relatives	4%	12%
Adoptive parents and adoptive siblings	4%	3%
Biological half-siblings (total sample)	3%	16%
Biological half-siblings (paternal only)	3%	18%

From Kety et al., 1976

disorder. Yet environmental factors also contribute to onset of the disorder. How does the investigator determine the relative contribution of heredity and environment. To this point, the methods described suggest whether or not heredity contributes rather than the degree to which heredity contributes. The methods assume, except in cases of full penetrance of disorders transmitted via Mendelian patterns (such as Huntington's disease), that the environment also contributes, but they do not assess the relative contribution of each. Quantitative studies of heritability help determine the relative contribution of each.

QUANTITATIVE STUDIES OF HERITABILITY

Most psychiatric disorders are thought to be inherited multifactorially—i.e., the inheritance of the disorder is governed by many genes. With multifactorial inheritance, the frequency distribution of the disorder in the population tends to fit a bell-shaped curve, albeit one that is skewed (see Figure 11–2c). Therefore, quantitative genetic techniques have been instituted in order to estimate the degree to which the disorder can be attributed to heredity rather than visually exploring pedigrees to determine Mendelian inheritance, as in the Egeland study.

In Figure 11–2, the distribution in the population of a characteristic is illustrated. If this trait is determined by a single gene with two alleles, there are three distinct phenotypes (see Figure 11–2a). When one assumes two genes contribute to this trait, as seen in Figure 11–2b, the number of phenotypes increases to five. Adding more genes (Figure 11–2c) causes the distribution of phenotypes to begin to form a bell-shaped curve. The distribution of depressive symptoms in population studies, a skewed bell-shaped curve, suggests that more than one gene (as well as environmental factors) contributes to the expression of symptoms.

Population genetic studies enable an investigator to determine the fraction of the observed phenotypic difference in distribution observed in the sample which is caused by heredity. This approach to understanding hereditary and environmental contributions can be expressed in the following formula:

$$V_p = V_g + V_e$$

where the variance of a characteristic in the population (V_p) such as depressive symptoms is equal to the genetic variance (V_g) plus environmental variance (V_e). The overall heritability (the relative contribution of genetic factors to the observed behavior) is

$$\frac{V_g}{V_P}$$

or the genetic variance divided by the overall population variance. The environmental variance can be further divided into the environmental contribution shared with relatives and environmental contribution which is independent of relatives.

A study by Gatz and colleagues (1992) illustrates how this methodology can be applied. In this study, a frequently used scale to measure depressive symptoms, the Center for Epidemiologic Studies–Depression Scale (CES-D), was administered to 68 monozygotic and 161 dizygotic twin pairs reared apart and 114 identical and 138 dizygotic pairs reared together in Sweden. All of the twins were elderly. By assuming a multifactorial pattern of inheritance and using quantitative genetics techniques, the investigators estimated that genetic influences explained 16% of the variance in total symptom scores, nonshared environment explained 55% of the variances, and shared environment explained 27% of the variance. (The method for determining the contribution of shared and nonshared environmental contributors is described below.) An additional 2% of the variance was unexplained. Inheritance explained much less of the total variation in symptomatic complaints of depression among these older adult twins than environmental factors. In addition, the influence of family rearing (shared environment), thought to play a substantial role in early onset depression, was not as important as the unique life experiences (unshared environment) among the older persons in this study. The reader must remember that this was not a study of more severe major depression but rather the self-report of depressive symptoms (a continuous variable—see Chapters 3,12) in a population of older adult twins in Sweden.

How can the study of twins provide this type of information? Six assumptions are made when using the twin model in quantitative genetics. First, the total variance of the trait of interest is the same in identical and fraternal twins and does not differ from the general population. According to this assumption, there is no reason to believe that depressive symptoms are more frequent in identical twins overall than in fraternal twins, and there is no reason to believe that depression is more or less frequent in all twins than in the normal population. Depression in a single twin pair may be associated, however. A second assumption is that differences within pairs of identical twins can only be environmental. In other words, identical twins share the same genome, and therefore any genetic contribution to depression would be identical for dizygotic twins. Mutations could undermine this assumption, but generally this assumption can be accepted for twin studies of depressive symptoms. Third, environmental influences not shared are as likely to vary for monozygotic as for dizygotic twins. For example, twins reared apart (whether monozygotic or dizygotic) do not share the same environment, and therefore a risk factor for depression, such as the death of a parent, would be equally likely for monozygotic as for dizygotic twins. The fourth assumption is that differences between monozygotic and dizygotic twins are genetic. In other words, environmental influences should not vary for monozygotic vs. dizygotic twins reared together. This assumption may not be so easy to defend, given that monozygotic twins may be treated "differently" than dizygotic twins. A fifth assumption is that genetic covariance (that is, the degree to which twins vary in the same direction) for dizygotic twins is half that for monozygotic twins. This assumption follows from Mendelian genetics—i.e., dizygotic twins are like siblings and, on average, share 50% of the human genome with their co-twin. Finally, it is assumed that environmental influences as well as genetic influences can make family members similar.

Figure 11–4 illustrates these assumptions in a hypothetical study of anxiety among monozygotic and dizygotic twins—some who lived together and some who lived apart. Anxiety symptoms were correlated in 75% of the monozygotic twins and 50% of the dizygotic twins (a much higher correlation than usually found in twin studies, but useful as an illustration). Twenty-five percent of anxiety symptoms were not correlated in monozygotic twins. According to the assumptions stated above, the differences within pairs of monozygotic twins can only be due to environmental influences. These environmental influences are therefore called nonshared (or within-family) environmental differences.

It is also assumed that the nonshared environmental differences are the same for

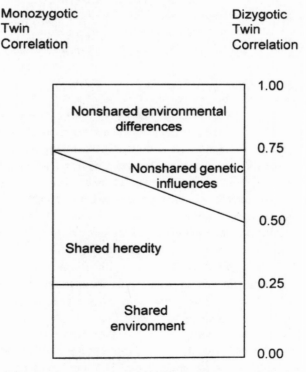

FIGURE 11–4. Hypothesized quantitative genetic study of twins to determine the relative contributors of heredity, shared environment, and nonshared environment to symptoms of anxiety. (Adapted from Plomin et al., 1990.)

monozygotic and dizygotic twins. Overall, monozygotic twins shared 75% of the variance: The anxiety scores were correlated at a .75 level. In contrast, dizygotic twins, overall, exhibit a correlation in anxiety scores of .50. The difference in correlation between .75 and .50 is considered the nonshared genetic influences (within-family genetic differences). The genetic variance between monozygotic and dizygotic twins was 50%, so the covariation between monozygotic twins secondary to heredity must be 50% and the covariance between dizygotic twins secondary to heredity must be 25%. Yet the monozygotic twins actually co-vary 75% of the time. How can we explain the difference? Twins (and other family members for that matter) also share environmental influences as well as genetic influences. Though shared (or between-family) environmental influences may be greater for twins than for nontwin siblings, this assumption is nevertheless applied in calculating environmental as well as hereditary contributions to the expression of psychopathologic symptoms such as anxiety. Therefore 25% of the similarity between the monozygotic and dizygotic twins was due to a shared (between-family) environmental influence. For most psychopathological conditions, environmental variance is due primarily to within-family influences, as illustrated in the study by Gatz et al. above.

The detailed statistical methods for calculating the relative contribution of hereditary and environmental influences are beyond the scope of this book. It is only necessary for the reader to recognize those data which must be obtained to calculate relative hereditary and environmental contributions to a disorder. In this case, it is necessary to obtain information regarding the zygosity of the twin pairs which are being studied and the psychopathological trait or disease of interest. By using multiple regression analysis (see Chapter 12), the contribution of shared environmental influences, nonshared environmental influences, and genetic influences can be calculated for the psychopathological trait. The procedures can be strengthened if the investigator has available information regarding whether the twins were reared together or apart.

Problem Set

Kendler and his colleagues (Kendler et al., 1992) performed a population genetics study using the assumption of multifactorial inheritance of depression and anxiety in order to determine the extent to which genetic factors were important in the etiology of major depression and generalized anxiety separately and to determine the shared and nonshared environmental contributions to each disorder. They also sought to determine to what extent the genetic contributions to depression and anxiety were shared. To perform this study, they interviewed 2,163 female twins from the population-based Virginia Twin Registry; all subjects were interviewed by someone "blind" to the psychopathologic states of the co-twin. Zygosity was determined by an algorithm based on questionnaire responses, photographs, and, where these sources were ambiguous, DNA polymorphisms. Five hundred ninety female monozygotic pairs and 440 female dizygotic pairs were studied. Diagnoses of depression and anxiety were determined by using *DSM-III-R* criteria for major depression and three definitions of generalized anxiety disorder (GAD): (1) duration of symptoms for at least 1 month and elimination of the *DSM-III-R* criterion that "the disturbance does not occur only during the course of a mood disorder"; (2) duration of the *DSM-III-R* symptoms of GAD for 1 month but the GAD could not occur during the course of a mood disorder; or (3) duration of GAD symptoms for 6 months but no requirement that the disturbance not occur only during the course of a mood disorder.

For the entire sample, the lifetime prevalence of major depression was 31.3%; the lifetime prevalence for 1 month GAD with or without mood disorder, 23.5%; 1-month prevalence of GAD without mood disorder, 16.7%; and 6-month prevalence of GAD with or without mood disorder, 5.9%. The proportions of the sample who had both lifetime major depression and each of the three GAD disorders were 16.2%, 9.3%, and 4.6%, respectively.

By applying quantitative genetic statistical techniques, Kendler and his colleagues determined that shared environment played no role in the etiology of either condition. Genetic factors were important for both major depression and generalized anxiety disorder: Over 50% of the variance was explained by heredity and between 47% and 31% of the variance, respectively, was explained by unshared environmental factors. The most interesting finding in this study was that heredity was not only an important contributor to both major depression and generalized anxiety: It was completely shared between the two disorders, suggesting that the genetic predisposition to major depression and generalized anxiety disorder among women is influenced by the same genetic factors, and therefore the vulnerability to either major depression or generalized anxiety results from their unshared environmental experiences.

Questions

1. This twin registry has been compiled over many years, but it does require voluntary participation in the registry. Do you think that volunteer participation may bias results of studies derived from the registry?

2. The average age of these twins was 30 years. What potential bias may result from the age of subjects?

3. The prevalence of major depression and generalized anxiety disorder (even lifetime diagnoses) is high in this sample. How can this be explained?

4. Were the methods for determining zygosity in this study adequate?

5. Are there, perhaps, other explanations for the striking finding that genetic factors were completely shared between major depression and generalized anxiety?

6. Why did the authors explore three different definitions of generalized anxiety disorder?

Answers

1. In general, the degree of bias from voluntary twin registries is probably acceptable. Twins who elect to participate in such registries are, naturally, more interested in issues regarding twins and therefore perhaps more interested in simi-

larities with their co-twin. (They may also be interested in differences from their co-twin.) Therefore, twins participating in a registry that is predominantly voluntary would potentially bias the sample toward twin pairs who share more characteristics, regardless of zygosity. Perhaps depressed twins who knew that their co-twin had also been depressed were more likely to participate and therefore biased the findings toward an estimate of greater hereditary contribution than is actually the case.

2. The age of onset of first episodes of major depression in women certainly extends well beyond 30 years of age. Therefore many women may develop depression at a later age and therefore be undiagnosed at the time the study was performed. Late-onset depressive episodes are thought to be less likely hereditary and therefore the hereditary contribution to the covariance would decrease. Longitudinal follow-up of the cohort will be essential. For example, in the Egeland linkage studies of manic-depressive illness, further diagnoses changed over time within the pedigrees and reduced the LOD scores. Therefore the initial positive findings of linkage proved not as strong as originally had been thought.

3. The authors recognized this as a problem and suggested that even though the prevalence figures were higher than those found in the Epidemiologic Catchment Area study, they were similar to or lower than those found in more recent population- based surveys. The lifetime rates of major depression among women in the National Comorbidity Study are similar to the rates in this study, yet that study covered women whose ages were between 18 and 54 years (and therefore one would expect an overall higher lifetime prevalence). The authors also noted that they used a "clinician-based instrument with added reminders to assist in long-term recall." Even so, close to 40% of this sample were diagnosed as having a genetically driven psychiatric disorder, somewhat counterintuitive to our general views regarding the frequency of inherited psychiatric disorders (especially by the age of 30).

4. Yes. These procedures were state of the art. If one wished to take a step further and "validate" the algorithm used by the investigators, they could select a subsample of individuals where zygosity was assigned according to the algorithm and test the subsample using DNA polymorphisms.

5. Major depression and generalized anxiety disorders share many symptom criteria, including tiredness, difficulty sleeping, and problems with concentration. The comorbidity of the two disorders (if in fact they are two disorders) is frequent. Some investigators question whether generalized anxiety disorder is a unique disorder. These results suggest that the genetic contribution to major depression and generalized anxiety is identical and that the environmental experiences of individuals with this hereditary predisposition "shape" the phenotype into that of generalized anxiety disorder and/or major depression.

6. The symptom criteria for generalized anxiety disorder have changed significantly from *DSM-III* to *DSM-IV*. While these criteria were changing from one edi-

tion of *DSM* to another (without adequate data to justify these changes), there remains considerable uncertainty in the psychiatric community regarding the diagnostic criteria for generalized anxiety disorder. Therefore, more than one definition seems justified.

REFERENCES

Allgulander C., Nowak J., Rice J. P. 1991. Psychopathology and treatment of 30,344 twins in Sweden: II. heritability estimates of psychiatric diagnosis and treatment in 12,884 twin pairs. *Acta Psychiatrica Scandinavica* 83: 12–15.

Bertelsen A., Harvald B., Hauge M. 1977. A Danish twin study of manic-depressive disorders. *British Journal of Psychiatry* 130: 330–351.

Egeland J.A., Hostetter A.M. 1983. Amish study, I: affective disorders among the Amish, 1976–1980. *American Journal of Psychiatry* 140: 56–61.

Egeland J.A., Gerhard D.S., Pauls D.S., Sussex J.N., Kidd K.K., Allan C.R., Hostetter A.M., Houseman D.E. 1987. Bipolar affective disorders linked to DNA markers on chromosome 11. *Nature* 325: 783–787.

Gatz M., Pedersen N.L., Plomin R., Nesselroade J.R., McClearn G.E. 1992. Importance of shared genes in shared environments for symptoms of depression in older adults. *Journal of Abnormal Psychology* 101: 701–708.

Kaprio J. 1994. Lessons from twin studies in Finland. *Annals of Medicine* 26: 135–139.

Kendler K.S., Heath A., Martin N.G., Eaves L.J. 1986. Symptoms of anxiety and depression in a volunteer twin population. The etiologic role of genetic and environmental factors. *Archives of General Psychiatry* 43: 213–221.

Kendler K.S., Neale M.C., Kessler R.C., Heath A.C., Eaves L.J. 1992. Major depression and generalized anxiety disorder: same genes, (partly) different environment? *Archives of General Psychiatry* 49: 716–722.

Kendler K.S., Walters E.E., Neale M.C., Kessler R.C., Heath A.C., Eaves L.J. 1995. The structure of the genetic and environmental risk factors for six major psychiatric disorders in women. Phobia, generalized anxiety disorder, panic disorder, bulimia, major depression, and alcoholism. *Archives of General Psychiatry* 52: 374–383.

Kety S.S., Rosenthal D., Wender P.H., Schulsinger F. 1976. Studies based on a total sample of adopted individuals and their relatives: why they were necessary, what they demonstrated and failed to demonstrate. *Schizophrenia Bulletin.* 2: 413–428.

Lykken D.T., Bouchard T.J. Jr., McGue M., Tellegen A. 1990. The Minnesota Twin Family Registry: some initial findings. *Acta Geneticae Medicae et Gemellogicae* 39: 35–70.

McGuffin P., Katz R., Watkins S., Rutherford J. 1996. A hospital-based twin register of the heritability of *DSM-IV* unipolar depression. *Archives of General Psychiatry* 53: 129–136.

Moldin S.O., Gottesman I.I. 1995. Population genetics in psychiatry. In *Comprehensive Textbook of Psychiatry/VI*, 6th ed., (eds. Kaplan H.I., Sadock B.J.), vol. 1, pp.144–155. Baltimore: Williams & Wilkins.

Page W.F. 1995. Annotation: the National Academy of Sciences–National Research Council Twin Registry. *American Journal of Public Health* 85: 617–618.

Plomin R., DeFries J.C., McClearn G.E. 1990. *Behavioral Genetics: A Primer,* 2nd ed. New York: W. H. Freeman.

Roy M.A., Neale M.C., Pedersen N.L., Mathe A.A., Kendler K.S. 1995. A twin study of generalized anxiety disorder and major depression. *Psychological Medicine* 25: 1037–1049.

Tambs K., Harris J.R., Magnus P. 1995. Sex-specific causal factors and effects of common environment for symptoms of anxiety and depression in twins. *Behavior Genetics* 25: 33–44.

Tsuang M.T., Lyons M.J., Eisen S.A., Goldberg J., True W., Lin N., Meyer J. M., Toomey R., Faraone S.V., Eaves L. 1996. Genetic influences on *DSM-III*-R drug abuse and dependence: a study of 3,372 twin pairs. *American Journal of Medical Genetics* 67: 473–477.

12

ANALYSIS OF CLINICAL AND COMMUNITY RESEARCH DATA

OBJECTIVES

- To recognize the properties of quantitative data which are relevant to statistical analysis.
- To choose the statistical procedure which is appropriate to the stated hypothesis and the available data.
- To evaluate the appropriateness of a specified model.
- To summarize and present statistical data in a form which communicates the findings of a study clearly and succinctly.

CASE EXAMPLE

Warner et al. (1995) used data from the National Comorbidity Study (NCS) to estimate drug use and drug dependence in the U. S. household population. The NCS was based on a sample of noninstitutionalized persons aged 15–54 from the 48 coterminous United States augmented by a supplemental sample of students living in campus housing ($n = 8,098$) (Kessler et al., 1994). The investigators were interested in the lifetime and 12-month prevalence of nonmedical use of and dependence on illegal drugs (marijuana / hashish, cocaine / crack, heroin, hallucinogens), prescription psychotropic drugs (sedatives, tranquilizers, stimulants, analgesics), and inhalants. The investigators collected data on demographic characteristics of the sample, including gender, race, education, marital status, geographical region, age, and urbanicity.

Many psychiatrists will read research reports and even analyze data without benefit of formal statistics coursework or access to statistical consultation. Some general analytic concepts are presented in this chapter to equip the clinician not well grounded in statistics to read, understand, and interpret many analysis plans and research results published in psychiatric journals and to collaborate knowledgeably with trained biostatisticians when the necessity arises.

How one analyzes clinical or community research data is determined by (1) the research hypotheses or questions, (2) the availability of data, and (3) the form of the available data. The research hypotheses or questions should describe clearly which exposures and outcomes the investigator is interested in and, in the case of an analytic study, what relationship among these factors is postulated (cf. Chapter 2). The study hypotheses (or questions) should be clear at the close of the paper's background and significance section because they set the stage for the methods section. In the case example, the reader learns at the end of the background section that NCS data would be used to calculate the prevalence and risk factors for drug use and dependence. Hypothesized etiologic relationships were not stated. If they had been stated, they might have taken the following form: "Age will be inversely associated with drug use," or "Male gender will be a risk factor for drug dependence."

The first part of the methods section describes the sample from which the data were collected. The second part of the methods section specifies how the exposure(s), outcome, and potential confounders are defined and operationalized, in other words, how all the *variables* are measured. A variable is any characteristic (for example, use of sedatives) that differs or varies from one subject or observation to the next. The final part of the methods section describes the analysis plan for examining the data. After reading a methods section, the reader should be able to identify (1) which constructs need to be measured, (2) how those constructs are operationalized as measurable variables, (3) how the variables were scaled, and (4) whether the proposed analysis plan is appropriate to those constructs, operations, and scaling.

In the case example, the materials and methods section described the NCS national sample, how diagnostic assessment was made, and which analysis procedures were employed. Drug use was measured on two levels (i.e., never vs. ever having tried at least one of a specific group of drugs at least one time, excluding "medical use"). "Nonmedical use" was defined, and prescription and illicit drugs included in each category were specified. Also, symptom criteria used to assign the diagnosis of lifetime dependence were specified. The methods section listed but did not describe how risk factors for drug use were measured (Table 12–1).

TABLE 12–1. Characteristics of National Comorbidity Survey (NCS) respondents compared with total U.S. population

CHARACTERISTIC	U.S., % (n = 65,244)	NCS, % (n = 8,098)	
		WEIGHTED	UNWEIGHTED
Sex			
M	49.1	49.5	47.5
F	50.9	50.5	52.5
Race			
White	75.0	75.3	75.1
Black	11.9	11.5	12.5
Hispanic	8.6	9.7	9.1
Other	4.5	3.5	3.3
Education (years)			
0–11	22.5	22.3	18.2
12	36.8	37.4	33.1
13–15	21.2	21.7	26.3
≥16	19.5	18.6	22.4
Marital Status			
Married	59.8	62.9	54.5
Separated, widowed, divorced	10.1	10.0	15.5
Never married	30.1	27.1	30.1
Region			
Northeast	20.0	20.2	19.2
Midwest	24.6	23.8	25.6
South	33.7	36.4	35.6
West	21.7	19.6	19.6
Age (years)			
15–24	25.5	24.7	21.8
25–34	30.8	30.1	32.4
35–44	25.9	27.1	27.7
45–54	17.8	18.1	18.1
Urbanicity			
Metropolitan	71.2	67.8	68.9
Other urban	8.1	7.5	6.5
Nonurban	20.7	24.7	24.6

Source: Warner et al., 1995, Table 1

Most of these risk factors were straightforward sociodemographic variables which required no explanation; the one exception was urbanicity, the definition of which was found in the results section. Survival analysis and logistic regression were the analytic procedures of choice for analyzing age of first drug use and the odds of each risk factor given a positive history of drug use.

TYPES OF DATA

A good research report lists which variables were measured and how, including the wording of any interview items or the scaling of any laboratory measures which were not immediately apparent. The most common analysis plans rely on numerical data. Numerical data are of three main types: nominal (or discrete), ordinal, and interval. The distinction among types of data is important because each type is appropriate only to certain types of statistical procedures.

Nominal data classify research subjects into discrete groups (or categories) which have no rank order among them. As can be seen in Table 12–1, several demographic characteristics in the case example were measured as nominal variables. Gender had two categories (male and female), marital status and urbanicity had three categories, and race/ethnicity and region each had four categories. Drug use and drug dependence were also scored as nominal data. Yes-or-no questions are binary or *dichotomous* (having two levels) variables, a subset of nominal data. Nominal data are assigned numeric values (e.g., no = 0 and yes = 1) for use in analysis but cannot be ordered on any dimension. For example, a measure of "region" may assign the values of 1–4 to persons residing in the Northeast, the Midwest, the South, and the West, respectively, but the regions have no quantitative rank relative to each other.

Ordinal data are considered categorical or discrete even though research subjects are ranked on a hierarchical scale. In the case example, education was scaled ordinally as 0–11 years, 12 years, 13–15 years, and ≥16 years, reflecting increasingly more advanced categories of educational achievement. The values of 1–4 assigned to these groups reflect rank but not equal intervals. A subject who scores 2 has more years of education than a subject who scores 1, but the difference in their years of education may not be equivalent to the difference in years of education for subjects scoring 3 and 4.

Interval data, on the other hand, rank research subjects on scales with intervals equidistant from each other. Age is a common interval-level variable. The age difference between subjects aged 2 and 3 is the same as the age difference between subjects who are 92 and 93. In Table 12–1, age is collapsed into four 10-year intervals for descriptive purposes. Also in this study, age of first drug use was measured in 5-year age intervals from 0–4 through 50–54. Subjects on any level of this variable are approximately the same distance (5 years in age) from those on the level below and above them. Warner and colleagues, therefore, could have measured duration and cumulative drug use and dependence as interval-level data. For example, duration of drug use in months or years or the cumulative dose of specific drugs would be interval-level measures of drug use.

Some data do not lend themselves to enumeration. These include extended opinions, anecdotes, or explanations in prose form. Such data may be obtained from a subject or an interviewer in response to an open-ended question, i.e., one without any specified response categories. Such data are called "qualitative data" although this term is sometimes applied to the type of data called nominal data above. Regardless of terminology, unstructured data are particularly useful when investigators are exploring a relatively unstudied phenomenon or need more detail to gain specificity. For example, the earliest descriptive study of "anticipatory grief" described a case of perplexing behaviors and cognitions related to the threatened death of a spouse (Lindemann, 1944). These qualitative data suggested constructs potentially pertinent to that phenomenon which were subsequently operationalized and quantified in follow-up studies (Clayton et al., 1973; Hays et al., 1994). In another example, early genetic studies of psychiatric disorders were based on case histories of family pedigree. (See Chapter 11 for a description of pedigree studies of affective disorders among the Amish by Egeland and Hostetter, 1983.) Unstructured qualitative data are also useful when quantitative methods have failed to explain adequately an extremely complex phenomenon. For example, scientists studying global self-ratings of health (shown to be robust and independent predictors of mortality and morbidity among subjects whose objective measures of health are very similar) are presently enriching structured interviews with open-ended questions designed to provide a more informative description of the factors aggregated in a subject's overall subjective assessment of his or her health status. Readers interested in the structured analysis of such qualitative data are referred to Feldman (1995). These data, however, are not subject to statistical analysis (nor need they be).

PREPARING DATA FOR ANALYSIS

Readying quantitative data for specific analyses is one of the most tedious but, nonetheless, most crucial tasks of data analysis. Data will usually have been entered into an electronic format and checked according to standardized protocols. Some of the common pitfalls in the preparation of data for specific analyses are described below.

Missing Data

Most data sets are incomplete in the sense that some subjects do not provide usable data for a few variables. This occurs for a variety of reasons in spite of the best efforts of interviewers and data abstractors. Subjects often *refuse* to divulge information about income, for example, because they consider it intrusive. They may consider a question too difficult to answer and respond that they *do not know*. Some questions are skipped because they are *not applicable* to a subject, e.g., date of death for surviving subjects or ambulation questions for amputees. Therefore, most variable scales will include options for scoring responses such as, "Skipped/ Not Applicable," "Don't Know," "Refused," or "Not Available," assigning numerical codes (e.g., 96, 97, 98, and 99) for subjects whose specific data are missing for the reasons mentioned above. Impatience to start the statistical analysis sometimes tempts novice investigators (and experienced ones, as well) to skip examination of the frequency distribution of a variable, including the frequency of missing data, resulting in distorted estimates of frequency and association.

Should subjects with any missing data be removed altogether from the effective sample being analyzed? This issue has generated a large literature which is beyond the scope of this text. Two strategies are often employed to manage missing data. Some investigators restrict their effective sample to persons with complete data. If this strategy is used, rejected and retained subjects should be compared, where possible, with respect to whatever nonmissing demographic or other information is available. When persons with missing data are omitted from analysis, the possible effects on the exposure–outcome relationship should be discussed.

A second strategy imputes or assigns "reasonable" values post hoc in place of missing values. Such imputations are based on other available data (e.g., a mean value may be calculated from those subjects without missing data, or a value may be predicted on the basis of other related but nonmissing variables). Imputed values should never be entered directly as part of the original data set; rather, a newly named variable should contain both real and imputed scores. When a new variable such as this is used when estimating effects of exposures on outcomes, mathematical adjustments to the estimates are possible which test whether one's score on the outcome variable is related to having missing data on the exposure variable. More in-depth description of imputation methods may be found in Kalton (1983) and Rubin (1987).

An appropriately conservative strategy to deal with missing data removes subjects with missing data on the dependent variable or the primary exposure variable(s). Researchers should address in the research report the possibility that such removal may bias the generalizability of their results. Control variables may be imputed, preferably by using increasingly sophisticated imputation methods as the proportion of missing values increases. In many papers, as with the case example, the investigators do not discuss their methods for handling missing data.

Weighting Data

Sometimes an analysis requires "weighting" (cf. Chapter 6). This occurs when a study is based on a nonrandom sample. A random sample of a population is not always feasible. Sometimes a subgroup in the population is of special interest but of small number, necessitating an "oversample" of that group in order to have sufficient variability in that subgroup. Sometimes selection of subjects involves rules for sampling several levels of a population, e.g., hospitals, then wards within hospitals, then patients within wards. Some populations, such as drug users, may be particularly susceptible to nonresponse. Even though a sample is not strictly random, investigators would like to be able to generalize from the sample to the larger population.

Concerned that refusal to participate in their study might be associated with psychiatric morbidity, the investigators in the Warner et al. study offered financial incentives to a random sample of initial nonresponders. Because the data collected from these nonresponders after financial inducement indicated higher rates of lifetime and current psychiatric disorders among nonresponders, the investigators calculated a nonresponse adjustment weight. Two other weights were also employed: one to adjust for variation in probabilities of selection within and between households and another to adjust the sample to the national population distribution of the 1989 U. S. National Health Interview Survey. The investigators incorporated these weights into their statistical tests, which weighted subjects differently depending on their probability of being chosen. When presenting results of weighted procedures, investigators should show clearly which data are weighted (as in Table 12–1) and explain the principles according to which the weights were used.

Collapsing Data

Depending on the hypothesis being tested, it may be necessary to "collapse" some variables into fewer categories than the original scales contained. In general, variables of interest should be measured at the highest level of specificity possible during data collection within the constraints on interview time and subject's memory. Subsequent to data collection, interval-level scales can always be collapsed into discrete categories, but discrete categories cannot be divided into more intervals than were used in the original measurement of the variable.

Sometimes data are collected as interval data and then reported as collapsed. The authors in the case example collected income and education data as interval-level data and then collapsed these data into ordinal-level subgroups. By doing so, they obscured the distribution of these variables in their sample, but that loss of information was offset by other advantages. Estimated odds associated with a finite number of conceptually meaningful risk categories are more useful to clinicians and health planners than estimated odds associated with each single-dollar increase in income or each single year of additional education. To this end, income was collapsed into four categories of $0–$19,000, $20,000–$34,000, $35,000–$69,000, and ≥$70,000, and education was collapsed with reference to commonly acknowledged educational milestones of high school and college achievement.

Nominal variables and ordinal scales, such as those described above, are often analyzed as *dummy variables* when the investigators wish to quantify increasing (or decreasing) levels of risk compared to a reference level. In the case example, odds of drug use across racial groups were calculated using a dummy variable for race where whites were treated as the reference group. Odds of drug use in other racial groups were compared pairwise with whites, i.e., black vs. white, Hispanic vs. white, other vs. white. Other reference groups shown in Table 12–2 include college graduates (compared to subjects with less education), subjects earning $70,000 or more (compared to less wealthy subgroups), Midwesterners (compared to subjects from other regions), and nonurban dwellers (compared to metropolitan and other urban.)

TABLE 12–2. Demographic correlates of lifetime drug use in the total sample and lifetime dependence among users

DEMOGRAPHIC CORRELATE	LIFETIME DEPENDENCE (USER SUBSAMPLE)	
	ODDS RATIO	95% CONFIDENCE INTERVAL
Race		
White	1.00	—
Black	.69	.46–1.03
Hispanic	1.05	.65–1.69
Other	.97	.39–2.42
Education (years)		
0–11	2.30[a]	1.60–3.29
12	1.69[a]	1.21–2.37
13–15	1.30	.88–1.91
≥16	1.00	—
Income (× $1,000)		
0–19	2.24[a]	1.43–3.52
20–34	1.51	.90–2.54
35–69	1.29	.76–2.21
≥70	1.00	—
Region		
Northeast	1.22	.86–1.71
Midwest	1.00	—
South	1.24	.89–1.73
West	1.64[a]	1.23–2.19
Urbanicity		
Metropolitan	1.40	.98–2.00
Other urban	1.38	.92–2.08
Nonurban	1.00	—

[a]An odds ratio with a confidence interval that does not include 1.0 is statistically significant

Source: Warner et al., 1995, Table 7

TYPES OF STATISTICS

Statistics are quantities derived from measures of a sample of a population. Statistics include all the ways that samples of a population are counted, described, and compared. Statistics can be descriptive or inferential.

Descriptive Statistics

Descriptive statistics describe the properties of the sample itself. Presenting descriptive statistics in analytic studies is important for at least two reasons. First, it permits the reader to evaluate which inferential statistics are appropriate to the data. (For a discussion of causal inference, cf. Chapter 1). Second, it permits results from more than one study of the same phenomenon to be compared, such that psychiatrists can assess the comparability between the described sample and patients in their clinical practices.

Common types of descriptive statistics are listed in Table 12–3. Descriptive statistics include simple frequency counts of subgroups of the sample (e.g., men and women, or subjects with and without a history of illicit drug use) as well as the proportion of such subgroups represented in the total sample. In most research papers, the first table displays descriptive statistics for the sample. Table 12–1 can be used to calculate the number of men in the sample: $n = 3,846$ (from the total $n = 8,098$ and the unweighted proportion 47.5%). These are descriptive statistics of the nominal-level variable, gender. Interval variables, on the other hand, are usually described by their properties of central tendency, including their average (or mean) value, the middle (median) value, and the most frequent value (or mode), as well as by their measures of variability, i.e., how the values on either side of the

---

TABLE 12–3. Common descriptive statistics

- Measures of classification
  Counts of category frequency and proportions of the whole

- Measures of central tendency
  Mean: arithmetic average $(\overline{X})$
  Median: middle score in a scale
  Mode: most frequent score in a scale

- Measures of variability
  Range: highest and lowest values of a scale
  Variance (v): sum of squared differences between each score and
      the sample mean, divided by the sample size minus 1
  Standard deviation (s.d.): square root of the variance
  Standard error (s.e.): average deviation of sample means from the
      population mean
  Interquartile range: the 2 values at the 25th and 75th percentile

---

average value are spread out. In the Warner et al. study, however, age data are presented only as frequency counts by 10-year age groups rather than using measures of central tendency and variability. Measures of variability include the range, the variance, the standard deviation, and the standard error. The *range* specifies only the highest and lowest value of the sample (for example, the age of the youngest and oldest subjects). The sample *variance*

$$\frac{\sum (X - \bar{X})^2}{n - 1}$$

(where Σ = sum, X = individual value, $\bar{X}$ = sample mean, and n = sample frequency) represents an overall measure of how each of the individual values for the subjects differs from the mean in the sample. Because differences between individual values and the mean are positive for values greater than the mean and negative for values less than the mean, the overall sum of these differences is equal to zero. For this reason, the variance is calculated as the sum of *squared* distances from the mean (divided by the sample size minus 1). Unfortunately, squaring yields a different unit of measurement than the original data. Therefore, taking the square root of the variance, the *standard deviation* (s.d.)

$$\sqrt{\frac{\sum (X - \bar{X})^2}{n - 1}}$$

represents a solution to this problem, because doing so yields the average distance between individual scores and the mean sample score in the same unit as the original data. The first standard deviation on either side of the mean score includes approximately 95% of the individual scores; two standard deviations includes 99% of the individual scores. Thus, if the mean ($\bar{X}$) age of a sample is 49, and the standard deviation (s.d.) is 7, then a 24-year-old in this sample is 2 standard deviations below its mean, i.e., one of the youngest persons in the study. In the same way that the standard deviation is a measure of how individual subjects scored with respect to the mean score in the sample, the *standard error* (s.e.) is a measure of how far the average sample mean is likely to have fallen from the true population mean if multiple samples were tested and their means were averaged.

In summary, when investigators provide the reader with a standard deviation, the reader has a measure of the variability in the particular sample tested. If a standard error is presented, the reader can begin to make inferences about how much variability there is in the entire population. The larger the sample size, the better will be its approximation to the normal distribution of the population. When interval data are not distributed approximately as a bell-shaped curve (i.e., with most persons scoring in the middle range and approximately equal numbers on either side of the centralized bulge of scores), the data are said to be "skewed" or non-normally distributed. For skewed data, variability can be assessed by presenting an interquartile range.

Inferential Statistics

Inferential statistics permit one to draw conclusions regarding a population from results observed in a sample. The principles underlying causal inference are discussed in more detail in Chapter 1. This chapter focuses on which inferential statistic or statistical procedure is appropriate to each type of data available. The calculation of each statistic and the discussion of assumptions underlying each test are beyond the scope of this text. Readers are urged to consult trained biostatisticians when developing their own research analysis plans.

Inferential statistics are available for studying the relationship between two variables (bivariate associations) or among many variables (multivariable associations). Common bivariate tests of association are summarized in Table 12–4. When both variables are nominal or ordinal, a chi-square statistic is usually appropriate. When one or both of the variables is interval, the choice of a statistical test depends on the shape of the frequency distribution of the variable(s) as well as on which one is nominal and which one is interval. Parametric tests are appropriate for interval-level variables whose scores are normally distributed in the sample. Where frequency distributions are severely skewed (i.e., non-normal), non-parametric tests are most appropriate. For example, depressive symptom scores in community samples are skewed toward the very low end of a frequency scale: most adults in a community report relatively few symptoms of depression whereas a small proportion of adults will report high numbers of symptoms. Because the majority of scores do not clump in the middle of the depression scale, a nonparametric test would be more appropriate for analyzing predictors of such scores.

TABLE 12–4. Common bivariate statistical tests

PARAMETRIC TEST	NONPARAMETRIC ANALOG	VARIABLE 1	VARIABLE 2
Chi-square test	—	Nominal or ordinal	Nominal or ordinal
Unpaired t-test	Wilcoxon rank sum	Binary	Interval
Paired t-test	Wilcoxon signed rank	Binary	Interval
One-way ANOVA	Kruskal-Wallis	Nominal or ordinal	Interval
Correlation coefficient (r)	Spearman's coefficient	Ordinal or interval	Ordinal or interval

However, in a sample of recently bereaved elderly subjects, depressive symptoms scores may be normally distributed, and parametric tests would therefore be appropriate.

The chi-square (χ^2) statistic tests the independence of two nominal or ordinal variables. For example, is drug use (positive lifetime history vs. negative lifetime history) independent of gender (male vs. female)? Chi-square tests are sometimes called contingency table tests because data are examined in the cells of a 2×2 (cross-tabulated) table. If the frequency of subjects in any cell is very small and might be expected by chance to fall below $n = 5$, Fisher's Exact Test is a more appropriate test of independence than the χ^2 statistic.

The unpaired t-statistic (sometimes called the two-sample t-statistic) tests for a difference in the mean scores of two independent groups. For example, are the mean ages of first drug use different among males and females? When the differences across three or more group means are tested, one-way analysis of variance (ANOVA) is used. For example, is the mean age of first drug use different among whites, blacks, and Hispanics? T-tests and ANOVAs examine the relationship between one interval variable and one nominal variable of two or more levels, respectively. When comparing mean scores of an interval variable whose frequency distribution is significantly non-normal, Wilcoxon rank sum and Kruskal-Wallis tests may be substituted for comparisons of two groups and three or more groups, respectively. For example, if the age of first onset were dramatically skewed toward the youngest age groups sampled, one of the nonparametric tests would be more appropriate than a parametric test.

In the case example, the investigators used a t-test for testing the independence of two binary variables (drug use and gender) where one would have expected a chi-square test of independence. The authors explain that the complex sampling design and extensive use of weights distorted the more typical estimates of the relationships. They also reference a published paper which describes the alternative use of a t-statistic to adjust for the distortion. The average reader, when faced with a less common statistical strategy, should expect a reasonable explanation for the strategy, including citation references, as provided in the case example.

The paired t-statistic tests for a difference in the mean score of two groups when the scores of the groups are not independent. For example, if the same sample of individuals was tested before and after an intervention, the paired t-statistic would test whether the change (or difference) in each set of paired scores averaged over all the individuals who participated was significantly different from 0. Also appropriate to the paired t-test are study designs which involve twins, studies of right- and left-handedness, and randomized assignment of subjects from a single population to two different interventions (because once subjects are chosen for intervention #1, being chosen for intervention #2 is not independent of having been chosen for intervention #1). The nonparametric analog for the paired t-statistic is the Wilcoxon signed rank test.

Pearson's r-statistic tests the correlation between two interval variables with approximately normal distributions. For example, are age of first drug use and years of education significantly related? If scores on each variable were plotted on a biaxial graph, the strongest correlations (r close to 1.00 or -1.00) would appear more like a straight line, and the weakest correlations (r close to 0.00) would appear as a round cloud of data points. Where the assumption of normality is not met for the two variables, Spearman's rank coefficient is the appropriate statistic.

Multivariable statistics are critical tools for the analysis of epidemiological data. Multivariable statistics permit the investigator to examine the relationship between an exposure and outcome while controlling for the confounding factors inevitably present in observational study designs. (The nature of confounding is discussed in greater detail in Chapter 7.) Multivariable statistics are also useful for examining the effects of an exposure on a disorder across levels of a third factor.

Multivariable statistics are derived from *mathematical models*. A multivariable model is a mathematical representation of proposed relationships among several variables. Multivariable statistics quantify those relationships. In recent years, the revolution in electronic computing has made possible an upsurge in the use of multivariable modeling. Unfortunately, the increased use of these techniques has not always been accompanied by the appropriate evaluation of assumptions underlying these procedures. General aspects of model structure relevant to the evaluation process, and some of the various types of models used, are reviewed below.

Often the goal of the psychiatric investigation is to explain the extent to which a disorder depends on variation in several exposure variables, i.e., a web of causation (see Chapter 1). For example, how much does drug dependence depend on age, gender, race, and income? In multivariable modeling, the disorder, in this case, drug dependence, is designated the *dependent variable*. The dependent variable is sometimes called the target or outcome variable. (Two or more dependent variables may be designated, although that is not the case in this example.) Exposure variables are called *independent variables*. Covariates (variables that change as the dependent and/or independent variables change) appear on the same side of the multivariable equation as independent variables. Dependent and independent variables and covariates may be nominal, ordinal, or interval. Their type, their distribution, and their hypothesized relationships determine which multivariable test is appropriate. Table 12–5 lists equations representative of common inferential models.

Logistic regression is used when the dependent variable is binary (e.g., when an outcome variable is the presence or absence of a *DSM-IV* diagnosis). Logistic regression models may include nominal, ordinal, or interval independent variables and may be adjusted for covariates. Warner and colleagues used simple logistic regression to study the association between several demographic characteristics and drug dependence. Their method is called *simple logistic regression* because the procedures were restricted to bivariate analyses only. Table 12–2 shows the results

TABLE 12–5. Common inferential models

STATISTICAL PROCEDURE	EQUATION[a]
Nominal outcomes	
Logistic regression (unadjusted univariate)	$M = A$
Logistic regression (adjusted multivariable)	$M = A\ B\ X1\ X2$
Event–time analysis	$M\ (\text{time}) = A\ B\ X1\ X2$
Ordinal outcomes	
Ordinal multinomial logistic regression	$N = A\ B\ X1\ X2$
Interval outcomes	
Simple regression	$Y = X1$
Multiple regression	$Y = X1\ X2\ A\ B$
One-way analysis of variance (ANOVA)	$Y = A$
Two-way analysis of variance	$Y = A\ B$
Analysis of covariance (ANCOVA)	$Y = X1\ A$
Multiple regression w/ polynomial	$Y = X1\ X2\ X2^2$
Multiple regression w/ product terms	$Y = X1\ X2\ (X1 \times X2)\ A\ B\ (A \times B)$
Multivariate regression	$Y1\ Z1 = X1\ A$
Multivariate ANOVA (repeated measures)	$Y1\ Y2 = X1\ A$

[a]M = nominal dependent variable; N = ordinal dependent variable; Y = interval dependent variable; $Z1$ = interval dependent variable; $Y1,Y2$ = interval dependent variable measured repeatedly; A,B = nominal or ordinal independent variables; $X1,X2$ = interval independent variables

of five simple logistic regression models. The dependent variable, lifetime history of drug dependence (among lifetime users only), was regressed separately on five ordinal independent variables: race, education, income, region, and urbanicity. Results are displayed as exposure odds ratios (cf. Chapter 8).

Two-way analysis of variance (ANOVA) is used when the dependent variable is interval, and the two exposures are nominal or ordinal. For example, age of first drug use might be regressed on gender and race in a two-way ANOVA. Simple and multiple regression (e.g., ordinary least squares [OLS] regression) and analyses of variance (ANOVA) and covariance (ANCOVA) are used when the dependent variable is interval and the exposures and covariates are nominal or interval or both. If the age of first use model above were expanded to include not only gender and race but also the subjects' age and income, then either OLS regression or ANCOVA procedures would be appropriate. Two-way ANOVA and ANCOVA are particularly useful when the main research question involves comparing the mean outcome scores across several treatment groups while controlling at the same time for baseline differences and randomization failures. Multiple regression is often used to develop broad-based models which specify multiple correlates or predictors of an outcome.

Multivariate analyses are a subset of multivariable analyses. Multivariate analyses employ two or more interval dependent variables. Independent variables and covariates may be either nominal or interval or both. One subset of multivariate

ANOVA is known as *repeated measures* ANOVA. Repeated measures tests are used to test whether subjects display different trajectories of repeated test scores over time. For example, a depressive symptoms inventory might be administered to spouses of both elective surgery patients and emergency surgery patients once at the beginning of the hospital experience and repeatedly at 6-week intervals for a total of five administrations. The spouse's five depression scores would become the five dependent variables. The exposure variable would be the type of stressor (elective vs. emergency surgery). Differences in repeated measures trajectories would be tested with an F-statistic.

Survival analysis (also known as event–time analysis) tests whether the timing of an event is dependent on variation in selected independent variables. In the case example of drug use, the authors tested whether the timing (in 5-year intervals from 0–4 years to 50–54 years) of an event (first use of drugs or first dependence on drugs) was dependent on an exposure (birth cohort). Other commonly studied events might include suicide, age of onset of a disorder, recurrence or remission of a disorder, or other discrete events. Survival analysis requires data collected over time (longitudinal), although the time period may have concluded at some time in the past (retrospective) or may continue to a specified time in the future (prospective). Once an event occurs to a subject, the subject cannot be counted again for a second event and is censored (i.e., dropped from the analysis). Subjects who die in the course of a study are censored. Another example of censoring can be found in the depression study described in Chapter 3; patients in this analysis who experienced recurrence of a major depressive episode were censored when this event occurred. Survival analyses can also take into account other kinds of subject loss besides the occurrence of the event itself, e.g., if a subject moves out of the tracking area or refuses to continue with the project. Survival analysis is a nonparametric test. It does not depend on a specified distribution of events over time. Differences in the timing of the event across exposure groups are tested with the Z-statistic.

Factor analysis is another multivariate procedure frequently used in psychiatric research for the construction of symptom rating scales, such as the Center for the Epidemiologic Study of Depression (CES-D) scale (Radloff, 1977) and the Beck Depression Inventory (BDI) (Beck, 1967). In this procedure, a large number of items representing, for example, depressive symptoms, are administered to a group of patients. A patient's score on each individual item is assumed to consist of one or more factors, i.e., latent, unobserved variables. Four factors have been reliably demonstrated from the 20-item CES-D scale: positive affect, negative affect, somatic complaints, and interpersonal problems (Ross and Mirowsky, 1984). Based on the scores of individual items, the factor analysis estimates factor loadings which indicate the importance of a specific factor for a given item. Knowledge of which factors load heavily on an item can assist investigators to select items for a scale that is parsimonious and covers all the dimensions of interest. Factor analysis and related procedures, such as discriminant function analysis and cluster analysis, are described more extensively in Kleinbaum et al. (1988).

Quantifying nonlinear effects

Sometimes the relationship between an exposure and an outcome is not linear. For example, drug use may increase as age increases, but only up to a certain age range, at which time drug use begins to decline as age increases further. This relationship between drug use and age would appear as a curve shaped like an inverted U. Nonlinear effects are best observed using a scatter plot of the exposure–outcome relationship. Observed nonlinear curves can be tested in statistical models by means of transformed terms of the exposure variable. Two examples of transformed terms are polynomials (e.g., squared or cubed variables) and logarithmic terms (e.g., the natural logarithm of the variable). Where a polynomial is included in a model, the respective simple linear term is usually included. In the case example, both age and age squared would be entered into a model of drug use. A complete discussion of modeling nonlinear relationships may be found in Kleinbaum et al. (1988).

Product terms

The effect of a single risk (exposure) factor on a disorder may also change across levels of a second factor. This phenomenon has been labeled an *interaction effect,* a *suppression* (or *potentiator*) *effect,* and an *effect modification.* Such an effect can occur when a risk factor is a predisposing, enabling, or reinforcing factor in the causal process of a disorder, as discussed in Chapter 1. Like curvilinear effects, effect modification is best examined using a combination of the following: (1) graphical displays of relationships, (2) stratified contingency (chi-square) tables or analyses of variance, and, if evidence of effect modification is suggested, (3) models which include a product term. A product term is constructed by multiplying the scores of two variables. Without the product term in the model, the estimated effect of an exposure variable represents its average effect across all levels of the covariate.

For example, it is well known that a stressful life event, such as a job loss, can be a precipitating factor (Paykel, 1994) for a major depressive episode (MDE). Similarly, a past history of multiple MDEs is also a predisposing risk factor for a future MDE. However, stressful life events may be less powerful risk factors as episodes of MD accumulate. Thus, in addition to the independent positive risk of MDE afforded by stressful life events and a history of multiple episodes as separate (main) effects, more frequent past episodes may mitigate (or suppress) the untoward effects of stressful life events when they are reported simultaneously by the patient because they interact with each other. One measures the statistical significance of such effect modification in a multivariable model of an outcome (e.g., recurrence) regressed over the two individual variables (e.g., stressful life events and past history of MDE) as individual (main effect) variables as well as on the interaction variable constructed from the product of these two variables (stressful life event × past history of MDE). If the product term is not included in the model, the observed effect of a stressful life event would reflect an average of its effect among patients who did and did not have a past history of an MDE.

The interpretation of a product term depends on the specific form of the model, i.e., the dependent variable. In the example above, where the dependent variable is dichotomous, the interactive effects of the two risk factors would be interpreted as multiplicative. This interpretation of a logistic regression model is most appropriate when studying the etiology of a disorder. Where public health concerns are paramount, the dependent variable is more appropriately tested in its continuous form, with multiple regression procedures, as discussed above. In this case, the interpretation of interaction is that the two factors are additive. For more detailed discussion of analytic strategy, the reader may wish to consult Kleinbaum et al. (1982).

SPECIFYING A MODEL

The number of possible multivariable models for specifying a particular exposure–disease relationship, given all the possible covariates, transformed terms, and product terms, is obviously too large to employ all models in the analysis. There is no best model, only relatively better and worse. A large literature—which is beyond the scope of this text—discusses how one selects better models. In general, one evaluates a model by asking, "Is the statistical procedure appropriate to the form of the variables, and are all relevant variables included in the model?" In Table 12–6, several more specific considerations for evaluating statistical models are summarized.

PRESENTATION OF ANALYZED DATA

Journal space comes at a high premium, and readers' time is precious. Author-investigators have the responsibility to describe their sample and related statistics in as clear and precise a way as possible. Readers should not have to search in vain for crucial information nor have to plow through more detail than is necessary. Choosing what to present and how to present it involves as much art as science. Prior to the development of tables or figures, the author must decide what is most relevant to include in the presentation. Table 12–7 lists some guidelines for embarking on these decisions.

The tables and figures from the paper by Warner et al. are generally helpful. Their tables are clear, although detailed, a result of needing to present additional data related to their complex weighting procedures. Figure 12–1 displays signifi-

TABLE 12–6. Evaluating choice of variables for a multivariable model

Does the choice of exposure variable(s) and confounders reflect what is known clinically about the correlates and etiologic agents of the outcome variable?
- How were potential confounders screened?
- What rules applied for including "true" confounders and excluding nonconfounders? (See discussion of confounding in Chapter 7.)
- How was the correlation among confounders and exposure(s) tested?
- How were the competing effects of correlated independent variables on the dependent variable resolved?

Were "stepwise" algorithms employed for model-fitting? Such algorithms begin with a small number of variables and add variables one at a time to determine how each addition changes the model (forward stepwise), or begin with all variables in the model and remove variables one by one (backward selection).
- If so, was the exposure variable always included in the model?
- Did the authors indicate that selection (or deletion) steps produced changes in estimates of effect which were incremental as opposed to varying in unpredictable ways?
- Was the underestimation of standard errors commonly associated with automated stepwise procedures addressed?
- If stepwise procedures were employed, was the criterion for retaining (or deleting) a variable stipulated and sufficiently conservative, i.e., $\geq 10\%$ difference in the estimated effect of the exposure?

Mathematical models are predicated on assumptions of an adequate sample to test for effects of an exposure on an outcome. Depending on the type of data (and modeling strategy), was the sample size sufficiently large to accommodate the number of variables in the model?
- For chi-square analyses using nominal data in a 2×2 table: were any expected cell counts < 5?
- For logistic regression analyses: were exposure and covariate subgroups > 5?
- For multiple regression analyses: was there at least one subject who could be categorized at each level of the exposure/covariate subgroups?

Was the adequacy of the regression model examined?
- What was the magnitude of the variation in the dependent variable that was not explained by the model (residual error)?
- What was the influence of extreme values (outliers) on any of the independent variables?

Were multiple procedures used to compare and contrast exposure and outcome groups?
- Graphs and figures
- Stratum-specific and/or summary measures based on contingency tables
- Simple models and models that adjust estimated effects for other variables

cant differences in the cohorts, but labeling (instead of numbering) the birth cohort results in the figure would have assisted the reader. In unpublished multivariable logistic regression models provided to the authors by Warner et al., the adjusted relationships were substantively different from the unadjusted relationships featured in the discussion section, so it is unclear why the unadjusted odds ratios

TABLE 12–7. Guidelines for presenting quantitative data

- *Consider your reader.* What statistical or methodological expertise or interest can be assumed of the reader? Will a clinical, research, or program planning perspective predominate among readers? The journal editor can be of great assistance on these points. Another help: Study representative tables and figures from the journal in question.

- *Annotate your tables such that they can stand alone.* Label your variables carefully to provide as much information about their scaling as the reader might need. Use footnotes and column headings generously to inform the reader about sample size, scaling of variables, and statistical procedures.

- *Make generous use of figures.* A picture is worth 1,000 words, particularly when demonstrating the meaning of transformed terms, product terms, and changes in exposures or course of disease over time.

- *Eliminate redundant or superfluous material.* Give the reader everything needed to calculate additional statistics of interest, but do not clutter a table with numbers which are unnecessary to inferential conclusions. Abundant white space around columns of numbers is more inviting to the eye than minimal white space.

- *Report your results in the order that your tables and figures are organized.* When explaining your tabulated findings in the text, proceed systematically from left to right and from top to bottom in your tables. Do not jump around to your favorite findings. Do not refer to unpresented analyses without noting that the data are not shown.

- *Report familiar epidemiologic measures.* For clinicians and policy makers who do not have an extensive statistics background, risk ratios and confidence intervals are of more utility and more intuitively accessible than are regression coefficients.

- *Present results for all hypotheses or research questions.* Explore thoroughly all relevant "loose ends." If one or more of your findings is perplexing or counterintuitive, perform additional subanalyses to understand the phenomenon better. Results of such analyses are often described only in the text, with a notation that the data are not shown. Readers expect that the analyses will be pushed to the limits of the data by the investigators since readers are unable to do so for themselves.

---

were presented in Table 12–2, when they could have been omitted. Inferences concerning racial differences in lifetime drug dependence and 12-month dependence based on unadjusted analyses were not supported in the adjusted model, which was omitted from the paper.

Problem Set

In a brief paper, Caton and colleagues (1995) noted that prior studies linking psychiatric disability with homelessness have not examined the 20% of homeless persons who are women. Previous studies of homelessness have found that "the homeless or residentially unstable have greater alcohol and/or drug abuse; higher symptom levels; greater non-compliance with prescribed treatments; and a greater prevalence of foster care, group home placement, and runaway episodes in childhood" (Caton et al.,

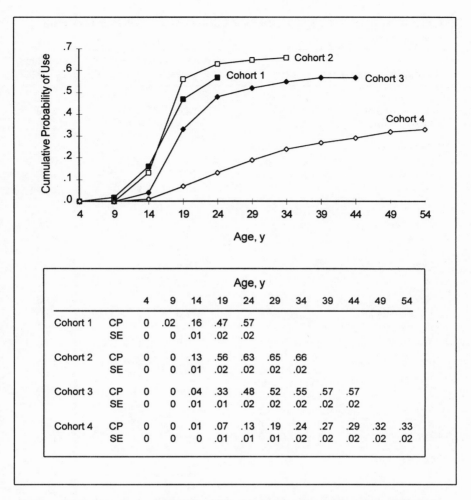

FIGURE 12–1. Cumulative probability (CP) of drug use, with standard errors (SE), in four cohorts of National Comorbidity Survey respondents. Cohort 1: ages 15–24; Cohort 2: ages 25–34; Cohort 3: ages 35–44; Cohort 4: ages 45–54. Redrawn from Figure 1 of Warner et al. (1995) in the same format.

1995, p. 1153). Their report replicates among women a previous study on schizophrenic men.

The dependent variable *literal homelessness* was defined as having "no fixed abode and (being) forced to sleep in the street or in the shelters" (Caton et al., 1994, p. 266). The exposure variables assessed three domains of risk factors: illness severity, family background, and prior mental health resource use and were measured with scales of known properties.

Potential confounders were controlled if they were related to homelessness at the p < .15 level (frequencies shown in Table 12–8). Ethnicity was the only potential con-

TABLE 12–8. Selected background characteristics of never-homeless and homeless women with schizophrenia

BACKGROUND CHARACTERISTICS	NEVER HOMELESS ($n = 100$), %	HOMELESS ($n = 100$), %
Place of birth		
American born	74.0	81.0
Foreign born	26.0	19.0
Race/ethnicity		
Black	39.0	52.0
Hispanic	26.0	10.0
White	35.0	38.0
Religion		
Protestant	32.0	40.0
Catholic	46.0	41.0
Other	13.0	15.0
None	9.0	4.0
Marital status		
Single	43.0	49.8
Married/conjugal	17.0	7.0
Separated/divorced	34.0	36.2
Widowed	6.0	8.0
Employment status		
Employed	21.0	26.0
Unemployed	79.0	74.0
Income from entitlements		
Yes	85.0	88.0
No	15.0	12.0
Earned income		
Yes	19.0	19.0
No	81.0	81.0
Income from family		
Yes	39.0	8.0
No	61.0	92.0
Current age (yr)		
Mean	43.0	42.0
Standard deviation	11.9	9.9
Years of education		
Mean	11.55	11.53
Standard deviation	2.95	2.10

From Caton et al., 1995, Table 1

founder related to homelessness. If ethnicity were also related to the risk factors, then the potential for confounding would be serious. However, the authors did not report tests of the relationship of ethnicity to the risk factors. Instead, all analyses were adjusted for ethnicity, although this was perhaps unnecessary. Income was not controlled due to its structural (rather than incidental) association with homelessness. The associations between risk factors and homelessness were tested with logistic regression models as shown in Table 12–9.

Based upon the findings shown, Caton and colleagues included the four risk factors significantly associated with homelessness (Table 12–9) in an untabled adjusted logistic regression model. Adequacy of family support was the only variable that demonstrated an excess effect: there were three times the odds of low family support among homeless urban schizophrenic women compared to urban schizophrenic women who were not homeless. In the final analysis (also untabled), the following stepwise logistic regression analysis of homelessness was performed to determine whether family support alone accounted for the effects of antisocial history and substance abuse:

- Step 1: Family support and ethnicity were forced into the model.
- Step 2: Antisocial history was added to the model in step 1; there were 10 times the odds of antisocial history among homeless women.
- Step 3: Alcohol and drug abuse were added to the model in step 2; neither demonstrated increases among the homeless.

In the companion article describing risk factors for homelessness among urban schizophrenic men, Caton et al. (1994), using an analysis which controlled for significant confounders such as immigration status, tenure in New York City, ethnicity, and veteran status, found that excess risk of homelessness among these men was associated only with drug abuse, inadequate family support, and having no long-term therapist.

Questions

1. What is the primary outcome of interest? How is it scaled?

2. How are the exposure domains operationalized? How are they scaled?

3. What potential confounders are examined (Table 12–8)? Which are nominal, ordinal, and interval? Which 'appear' to differ across the two homelessness groups?

4. Ninety-five percent of women in the study were within what age range?

5. From Table 12–8, give one or two examples of statistics which may have been used to test the differences in potentially confounding variables between the two groups.

6. Was logistic regression appropriate to testing the exposure–outcome relationship?

7. What other statistical tests would be appropriate for testing the simple (unadjusted) associations between homelessness and the risk factors? Among the alternative procedures, which do you believe has the greatest strategic advantage?

TABLE 12–9. Test of key hypotheses on the risk of homelessness among urban women with schizophrenia

RISK FACTOR	NEVER HOMELESS (n = 100)		HOMELESS (n = 100)		UNADJUSTED[a]		ADJUSTED[b]	
	MEAN	S.D.	MEAN	S.D.	LRT	p	LRT	p
Illness domain								
UCLA Social Attainment Scale score	19.3	7.1	20.4	7.4	1.10	.30	1.20	.27
PANSS Positive Symptoms score	15.4	6.5	16.5	7.7	1.22	.27	1.07	.30
PANSS Negative Symptoms score	17.6	7.3	18.9	6.5	1.66	.20	1.32	.25
Alcohol abuse (0=no, 1=yes)	.16	.37	.30	.46	5.60	<.05	5.61	<.05
Drug abuse (0=no, 1=yes)	.15	.36	.29	.46	5.79	<.05	5.39	<.05
Antisocial personality disorder (0=no, 1=yes)	.01	.10	.08	.27	6.45	<.05	7.03	<.05
Family domain								
Index of family disorganization	13.1	3.8	13.1	3.9	.00	.98	.15	.69
Adequacy of family support	1.8	1.1	2.6	1.3	18.06	<.01	12.96	<.01
Service use domain								
Medication adherence	1.64	.95	1.57	.95	.29	.59	.53	.46
Long-term therapist	49.4	51.9	39.6	54.4	1.51	.22	1.00	.32

[a]Likelihood ratio test (LRT) and p from logistic regression models with no other variables held constant

[b]Likelihood ratio test (LRT) and p from logistic regression models holding race/ethnicity constant

From Caton et al., 1995, Table 2

8. Suggest an exposure which might affect homelessness differently at different levels of a sociodemographic variable. How would you test effect modification?

9. In what way was the risk of homelessness among schizophrenic women obscured in the model containing the full set of four variables? How was it illuminated in the stepwise model?

10. Was the sample size adequate to the size of the models?

11. Is long-term therapy more protective against homelessness among men than among women?

Answers

1. Literal homelessness, scaled dichotomously.

2. The *illness* domain is operationalized with three interval variables: social attainment, positive symptoms and negative symptoms, measured with the UCLA Social Attainment Scale and the Positive and Negative Syndrome Scale (PANSS). The *illness* domain is further operationalized with three dichotomous items measuring substance abuse and antisocial personality from the SCID and SCID-II. The *family* domain is operationalized with two interval variables: family disorganization and adequacy of family support, measured with the Community Care Schedule and a scale of unknown properties described in detail in a footnote. The *service use* domain is operationalized as medication adherence and number of months with the same therapist, from the Community Care Schedule.

3. Potential confounders measured as nominal variables include place of birth, race, religion, marital status, employment status, income from entitlements, earned income, and income from family. Two potential confounders were measured as interval variables, including age and years of education. The most striking differences between the homeless and the never homeless are in racial subgroups and in income from family.

4. In this study 95% of the homeless subjects were between the ages of 32 and 52.

5. Chi-square statistics would be most appropriate for testing the independence of homelessness and nominal characteristics of the sample, e.g., place of birth, religion, or employment status. T-tests (or analyses of variance) were likely used to test for differences in the mean age or education of cases and controls, particularly if these variables demonstrated a generally normal distribution. Alternatively, the Wilcoxon Rank Sum score could have been used.

6. Logistic regression is appropriate to dependent variables which are dichotomous (homeless vs. never homeless).

7. Two alternatives for assessing the simple association of an exposure and the outcome include (1) an unpaired t-test of the differences in the means of interval variables in cases and controls (e.g., PANSS scores) and (2) a chi-square test of the independence of homelessness and nominal variables (e.g., alcohol abuse). The

advantage of the logistic regression model is that the simple association of exposure and outcome can be adjusted for important confounders of that association
(e.g., race/ethnicity).

8. Inadequate family support might be a more powerful correlate of homelessness among older schizophrenic women in particular. Older schizophrenic women
may have fewer social resources (e.g., parents) to contribute to residential stabilization. One might graph the level of family support by age group separately for
homeless and nonhomeless women. If there was evidence of a differential effect
among homeless and residentially stable women, then one would test this hypothesis with a product term (adequacy of family support × age) added to a model of
the main effects of these two variables on the probability of homelessness.

9. Full models describe the effect of an exposure on an outcome, taking into account the effects of all other independent variables together. Full models obscure
the impact of individual risk factors on the strength of association of other risk factors on the estimated exposure outcome. Careful stepwise building of models can
illuminate these changing effects. The authors of this example wondered whether
inadequate family support was by itself sufficient to explain the effects of antisocial history, alcohol abuse, and drug abuse, which had been observed in unadjusted analyses. By adding these variables in a stepwise sequence, Caton et al. observed that both inadequate family support and antisocial history had unique
effects on homelessness; substance abuse did not. Thus, interventions targeting
both family support structures and antisocial disorder may have a positive impact
on homelessness.

10. The fullest model tested included five exposures and one covariate. Such a
model would typically require at least 60 subjects (10 for each variable). Two hundred subjects is adequate to the specified model.

11. Long-term therapy reportedly reduced the odds of homelessness significantly among men but not among women. The statistical significance of the protective effect among men compared to among women could only be tested with a
data set which included both men and women. The appropriate logistic regression
model to test this interaction of long-term therapy with gender would regress the
measure of homelessness on at least three independent variables: gender, long-
term therapy, and the product term of gender × long-term therapy. The significance of the product term is the test of an increased protective effect of long-term
therapy against homelessness among men compared to among women.

REFERENCES

Beck A.T. 1967. *Depression: Causes and Treatment.* Philadelphia: University of Philadel-
     phia Press.
Caton C. L. M., Shrout P. E., Dominguez B., Eagle P. F., Opler L. A., Cournos F. 1995. Risk

factors for homelessness among women with schizophrenia. *American Journal of Public Health* 85: 1153–1156.

Caton C. L. M., Shrout P. E., Eagle P. F., Opler L. A., Cournos F. 1994. Risk factors for homelessness among schizophrenic men: a case-control study. *American Journal of Public Health* 84: 265–270.

Clayton P. J., Halikas J., Maurice W., Robins E. 1973. Anticipatory grief and widowhood. *British Journal of Psychiatry* 122: 47–51.

Egeland J.A., Hostetter A.M. 1983. Amish Study, I: affective disorders among the Amish, 1976–80. *American Journal of Psychiatry* 140: 56–61.

Feldman M. G. 1995. *Strategies for Interpreting Qualitative Data.* Qualitative Research Methods Series, Vol. 33. Thousand Oaks, CA: Sage.

Hays J. C., Kasl S. V., Jacobs S. C. 1994. The course of psychological distress following threatened and actual conjugal bereavement. *Psychological Medicine* 24: 917–927.

Kalton G. 1983. *Compensating for Missing Survey Data.* Research Report Series, Survey Research Center, Institute for Social Research. Ann Arbor: University of Michigan.

Kessler R. C., McGonagle K. A., Zhao S., Nelson C. B., Hughes M., Eshleman S., Wittchen H.-U., Kendler K. S. 1994. Lifetime and 12-month prevalence of DSM-III-R psychiatric disorders in the United States: results from the National Comorbidity Survey. *Archives of General Psychiatry* 51: 8–19.

Kleinbaum D. G., Kupper L. L., Morgenstern H. 1982. *Epidemiologic Research: Principles and Quantitative Methods.* New York: Van Nostrand Reinhold.

Kleinbaum D. G., Kupper L. L., Muller K. E. 1988. *Applied Regression Analysis and Other Mathematical Methods,* 2nd ed. Boston: PWS-Kent.

Lindemann E. 1944. Symptomatology and management of acute grief. *American Journal of Psychiatry* 101: 141–148.

Paykel E. S. 1994. Life events, social support and depression. *Acta Psychiatrica Scandinavica (Suppl.* 377): 50–58.

Radloff L. S. 1977. The CES-D Scale: a self-report depression scale for research in the general population. *Applied Psychological Measures* 1: 385–401.

Ross C. E., Mirowsky J. 1984. Components of depressed mood in married men and women: the Center for Epidemiologic Studies Depression Scale. *American Journal of Epidemiology* 119: 997–1004.

Rubin D. B. 1987. *Multiple Imputation for Nonresponse in Surveys.* New York: Wiley.

Warner L. A., Kessler R. C., Hughes M., Anthony J., Nelson C. B. 1995. Prevalence and correlates of drug use and dependence in the United States. *Archives of General Psychiatry* 52: 219–229.

RECOMMENDED STATISTICAL TEXTS

Gonick L., Smith W. 1993. *The Cartoon Guide to Statistics.* New York: HarperPerennial.

Leaverton P. E. 1995. *A Review of Biostatistics: A Program for Self-Instruction,* 5th ed. New York: Little, Brown.

Streiner N. 1986. *PDQ Statistics.* Toronto: B. C. Decker.

Wassertheil-Smoller S. 1995. *Biostatistics and Epidemiology: A Primer for Health Professionals,* 2nd ed. New York: Springer-Verlag.

INDEX